HOW MARIJUANA CURES CANCER

By

Joan Bello, M.S.

LIFESERVICES PRESS, INC.
SUSQUEHANNA, PA 18847

HOW MARIJUANA CURES CANCER

© Copyright 2012 by Joan Bello

Published by LIFESERVICES PRESS, INC
POB 61
SUSQUEHANNA, PENNSYLVANIA 18847

http://www.benefitsofmarijuana.com

LCCN: 2011916891
ISBN - 978-1- 4663304-9-8
Printed in the USA

TABLE OF CONTENTS

PART III

Abstract:

Marijuana Therapy *restarts intricate bio-chemical cellular anti-cancerous interactions that are automatic, sequential and simultaneous in the healthy organism and which have become degraded by system failure. Homeostatic control of these complex processes is mediated through The Cannabinoid System, a pervasive network of chemicals and receptors throughout the body that operates in an understated, anticipatory fashion in the arena of challenge to the organism from both within and without for the explicit purpose of dynamic balance. Science has determined that The Cannabinoid System itself becomes deficient in its regulatory function which allows for the expression of cancer. Stringent research over the last decade has proven that cannabinoids of the Cannabis Sativa Plant are efficient and safe restorative agents for the dysregulated Cannabinoid System. To exploit the potential curative actions of these phyto-chemicals in service of the profit motive, billions of dollars in research and development are spent each year as Big Pharma synthesizes one after the other of the over 80 known exogenous cannabinoids, attempting to simulate the efficacy of the intact plant and its synergistic permutations of nearly 500 compounds.*

This presentation *addresses long-term deficiency in The Breath as the originating cause of Cannabinoid System failure and particularizes the philosophy of Holistic Science as it relates to the Cancer Biopathy and its prevention and/or its dissolution by Marijuana Therapy. The observable, intricate details of the cellular benefits of marijuana as the natural outgrowth of sufficiency in the pattern of the breath, which sets the stage for a higher order of health and awareness are explained for the lay audience with the specific purpose of exposing the truth. In reference to the unique botanical aspects of Cannabis Sativa, it is hypothesized that the superior tolerance of cannabinoids to radiant UV-B rays may be integral to its unparalleled healing ability.*

References, Terms, Definitions, Disclaimers

The Benefits of Marijuana by Joan Bello documents many references in this work.

Marijuana and Medicine: Assessing the Science Base by Institute of Medicine (IOM): (1999) is referenced.

Biopathy Defined: What is Cancer? Traditional medical science views cancer as an invasion/tumor arising spontaneously in an otherwise healthy organism. In contrast, Wilhelm Reich defined cancer as *a systemic deficiency that progresses to putrefaction of the body due to chronic suffocation of the cancerous tissue.*

Marijuana/Cannabis/Cannabis Sativa: refers to intact fruit of the plant in contrast to extraction of molecules or synthetic versions of molecules.

Marijuana - historically coined as a **derogatory/racist** word. As such it is used purposefully to raise it from its political belittlement to the exaltation it deserves.

Marijuana Therapy: Employment of Cannabis Sativa to restore the dysregulation of The Cannabinoid System.

Disclaimer: Some cancers are suffocation of the organism via intolerable environmental damage that even the healthiest organism could not overcome. This presentation, however, speaks to those exposed to the same unhealthy milieu, some of whom succumb owing to an individual state of diminished being while others are able to ward off the commonplace hazards.

NB: Health in the Pattern of The Breath defines an organism with adequate mobility, appropriate nutrition, resting and thinking, since full, deep, smooth and silent breathing is not expressed in a nutritionally deficient, sedentary, unwholesome or anxious mode of being.

HOW MARIJUANA CURES CANCER

Author's Preface

This very long article or very short book was envisioned originally as a quick work that would explain very simply how the compounds of the *Cannabis Sativa Plant Cure Cancer.* The evidence has actually been around for quite some time although a satisfactory explanation of how the interface of Marijuana with the human body could actually cure cancer was not forthcoming. Indeed, scientific proof was mostly hidden for the past thirty years and hardly reported to anyone but a small group of interested scientists and activists.

As I tried to integrate what hundreds of studies were showing in isolated but stunningly complementary research that were proving beyond doubt very definite and specific curative properties of the compounds of Cannabis for all types of cancers, the short explanation took on a life of its own. In addition, it was necessary to make clear that there is far more to how Marijuana impacts and heals the whole person than what is seen in the test tube.

From the perspective of Holistic Science, *disease is understood as an energetic imbalance on a continuum of wellness* which is not in any way limited to what is visible under the microscope. In order for the lay audience to appreciate the profound healing potential within the ancient Cannabis Sativa, the holistic orientation as it views the physical, psychological and spiritual interface has been included.

While I gathered all the relevant benefits of Marijuana for the cancer patient, the article just kept growing. However, in the service of the world of text messaging and sound bytes, **every subject is indexed so that anyone who chooses not to read the entire book will be able to locate specific topics of interest.** This work was however conceived and written as a whole piece with the intention of sharing with the reader the full extent of the way Marijuana enhances all levels of human experience.

The presentation on the following pages is set out in Four Parts, any of which can be read on its own. There is some intentional over-lapping in explanations, facts and ideas, reframed however from another perspective to emphasize their importance as well as to adhere to the plan that the book can be read in separate but intelligible pieces. Whatever scientific terms are included hopefully are clear enough so that, with just a bit of focus, the non-professional will be able to appreciate how Marijuana allows for healing from the Cancer Biopathy.

Finally, I would like to address the research being conducted by a group of young, progressive and brilliant scientists who are attracted to the unique, versatile and timeless healing compounds of this ancient plant. Many of their studies prove that cancer is just one of many very serious conditions that Marijuana affects safely and with amazingly positive results. To them may I say: thank you! As you continue on with further research, it is my absolute firm intuitive knowledge that whatever physical, mental or even spiritual distress investigated with Cannabis as the remedy, will demonstrate benefits beyond anything so far envisioned, even by me. (2011)

Cancer is the Ultimate Imbalance.
Cancer is Anti-Life.
Cancer Cells Cannot Cooperate.
Cancer Inflames.
Cancer Destroys.

Introduction

The Hidden Knowledge:
Within the scientific community, there is no doubt that the chemical compounds in Marijuana cure cancer. Anticancer effects of Marijuana have been reported in dribs and drabs over the course of the last half century in international Medical Journals that are inaccessible to the public. Breast, Prostate, Brain and even Lung cancers have all responded positively to Marijuana Therapy. In fact, the latest, most stringent science suggests that the unique compounds of Cannabis Sativa (*phyto-cannabinoids*) can and often do *prevent cancer*. Nevertheless, among the less-informed majority, there is great confusion. Misinformation about Cannabis is everywhere. The actual facts are almost nowhere. This presentation seeks to disabuse the general community of its misperceptions and fears concerning the basic effect of Marijuana as well as to elucidate the curative benefit of the ancient plant specific to cancer (especially warranted to dispel the propaganda that suggests the contrary). (*The agenda responsible for purposefully distorting and hiding the truth about Marijuana for the last 75 years will not be addressed, except to acknowledge its source as the persistent periodic resurfacing down through the ages of unconscious misanthropes whose self-serving actions had/have dire consequences for all the creatures of the earth.*)

The Cancer Mystery:
Cancer is the most feared word a doctor can utter. It conjures up the image of long-term pain and suffering, bad luck, and even guilt. Although there are many carcinogens in modern life, the estimate that 40% of cancer is preventable through changes in life-style causes many victims to blame themselves. Yet hardly anyone knows what *cancer* really means. Despite the sophisticated statistics, theories and billions of dollars spent on research every year, who gets cancer and why is still a mystery.

Various agents cause cancer in some vulnerable populations but the basic vulnerability is not clear. People who eat "properly," do not smoke tobacco, exercise regularly and are not exposed to carcinogenic agents still develop cancer, while smoking tobacco, poor eating and unhealthy settings are often endured throughout a long lifetime with nary a problem. Notwithstanding that the statistics point solidly to vice and excess as high risk factors for developing the dread disease, nevertheless, those persons who endure the worst conditions / lifestyles without disease represent a population that needs be explained.

Failed Understanding of Conventional Medicine:
Symptom-based medicine is not concerned with this paradox. Causal relationships are considered irrelevant in the battle against an invasive and random enemy to be eradicated at all costs. *The battlefield is the patient.* Standard procedures range from *not-quite* lethal doses of concentrated poisons ("chemo"), to burning out diseased tissue ("radiation") and including surgical incising of any malignant mass, all at great cost to the victim (physically, mentally and financially). Conventional treatments are traumatic and debilitating to the body and horrifying to the mind, destabilizing yet further the already grossly imbalanced organism (*and outrageously do not contribute to curing the source of the cancer*).

In modern *allopathic* medicine, there is no ferreting out the **root cause**, no orientation toward whole-person health or how that pertains to the Cancer Syndrome and definitely no interest whatsoever in any cure effected by a natural plant. Nature is replaced by the laboratory. The mindset is one-pointed against the enemy which is viewed as random and unfortunate and perhaps related to vague unhealthy habits, but in the practical reality of the world of the cancer patient, in fact, cancer is dark, unknown and misunderstood.

It does wax strange that among the thousands of medical specialists, there does not seem to be any academically motivated collective curiosity as to how the intact, ancient and complex Marijuana compounds help to alleviate the symptoms of cancer; or what inherent quality of Marijuana actually diminishes the instances of cancer in the general population; or how marijuana can possibly cure cancers already progressed to the danger level. Into this contemporary arena of disregard and even disdain for time-tested natural medical wisdom, the strange reality has materialized that it is the stringent research of Western technological science itself that has proven beyond any doubt, that Marijuana is in fact, the **only safe and sure remedy** for cancer so far discovered. Indeed, it is the only therapy that has been shown to be completely anti-cancer!

It is sad and immoral but completely understandable that results of thousands of studies displaying the promise of natural Cannabis Sativa for reversing the Cancer Biopathy have not been reported to the lay population. It is criminal that these facts have been hidden and intentionally distorted, while behind the scenes Drug Companies conduct multi-million dollar research to put isolated single-molecule pieces (or copies) of Marijuana in a pill! for which a doctor can then write an expensive prescription that is not nearly as effective or as safe as the intact plant.

Whatever **Causes Cancer is Cloaked in Ignorance.**
That **Marijuana Cures Cancer is Hidden by Propaganda.**
How **Marijuana Cures Cancer is Not Known**

PART I

Holistic Health * Breath * Marijuana

The Holistic Understanding:
Holistic Health and Alternative Medicine" are names given to the translation of Eastern medicine into contemporary culture which views the human being as a highly organized containment of energy with physical, mental and spiritual aspects. The heaviest or gross energy of the body, the finer energy of the mind, and the highest vibration of the spirit are different facets of the same entity. Disruption in the energetic flux that courses through (and around) the body results in dis-ease and is therefore *expressive of* not *different from* the individual. No blame can be conferred however, for without knowledge of what is disordered and how to restore whatever it is, the unconscious behavior that results in the specific dysfunction cannot be changed. Cancer is merely a visible, concrete confirmation of long-standing distortion in the energy matrix that powers an individual life. If delivery of the energy is sufficiently deficient, over time, the underperformance progresses to cellular disorganization (such as a tumor) i.e., Cancer. The location, duration and strength of the insufficiency determine how the disease presents and progresses.

The Vibrational Effect:
Esoteric Traditions recognize the individual spirit as a closed circuit vibratory pattern that is the backdrop for the unique expression of each person. Many practices have been perfected over the course of millennia for the specific purpose of refining the invisible pulsing of the individual. Unobstructed delivery of the imperceptible energy is *Health* while continuous infusion of the finest energy is *Optimal Health*. Altered consciousness is the reception and registration of energy that is finer than usual. It is at this subtle level of life that Marijuana provides fundamental healing.

Merging of the encapsulated radiant energy of Cannabis Sativa with the invisible vibratory essence of a person has effects unimagined by objective science. But in an ironic twist of karma, the technical expertise of modern science itself has proven the visible and measureable synergy between the countless compounds of Marijuana and the physical, psychological and spiritual elements that comprise the person.

Marijuana Therapy Feared:
Successful Marijuana Therapy produces *higher* order functioning at the physical level as well as noticeable expansion/enhancement of thought. This is the *high* that is so denigrated and feared by materialism because it is alteration to a consciousness that embraces community rather than competition. Being concerned with others, displaying creative ideas, seeking more humane answers suggests *a sharing and caring* that is not compatible with capitalistic greed. But it is a healthy state to be in and has been coined as *"a good mood consciousness that might itself be curative"* according to the long term study of the Institute of Medicine.

Breathing Energizes the Organism:
The distinctive way a person breathes every day is the single factor most responsible for the quality of the entire life experience. Nothing contributes more to how one thinks, feels and acts than the unique nuances in the *pattern of the breath*. Eastern disciplines teach that disease results from habitual inadequacy in the process of breathing. To the extent that distress exists in the mechanism and/or the method of respiration is there an associated energetic dysfunction in some area/region of the entity. Disease defines the area of unconscious neglect wherein the habit of the breath is inadequate in supplying the requirement of the organism to maintain homeostasis. Conversely, optimum health is distribution of rich energy throughout the whole organism.

Research proves uncanny synergy between Cannabis compounds and body-chemistry that enhances all autonomic (automatic) function especially the *Pattern of the Breath*. Marijuana has a unique dual opposing action of operation that is completely compatible with the physiology of the balancing system of the human organism. Marijuana is a stimulant and a relaxant at the same time which is the reason: it is so safe; it operates differently for different people depending on their circumstances and state of being; it balances the entire organism thereby encouraging the curative process for so many diseases; and most importantly; it automatically enhances the natural breath!

The most noticeable, notable, immediate and far-reaching *Benefit of Marijuana* is enhancement of the breathing process from which naturally proceeds *Superior Healing* and *Optimum Health*.

The Marijuana Effect **Resettles the Organism**:
Through the superior nourishing that accompanies marijuana by enhancing depth, smoothness, rhythm and ease of breathing, an integration of autonomic processes occurs. With finer fueling and increased delivery, the individual is vitalized with serenity. Tensions vanish. According to every respectable study that has examined its effects (U.S. and internationally), there is no doubt that Marijuana is a natural balancing agent that works through intricate physiological processes to "modulate," "regulate" and "moderate" (again from the prestigious Institute of Medicine) the extremes of body chemistry that too often invite chronic and/or life-threatening disease. Chronic disease, such as The Cancer Biopathy, is the expression of long-standing disruption, distortion and diminishment in the energy flow which reflects (and exacerbates) disequilibrium in the mind and the body. Cancer is end stage consequence of such a disturbance. Marijuana dissolves the imbalance.

The Effects of Marijuana are Not at all Mysterious. They are However Quite Miraculous.

Limited Breath: (Disorder of the Life Experience)
The human entity is at once infinitely complex when viewed from the vast and complicated interconnections needed for smooth functioning but decidedly simple from the one-pointed measure of its ultimate aim of survival. In the vibrant and essential processes of a healthy person, each of the billions of cells in the body continuously breathes fully and with ease - unless threatened. The cooperative striving of all systems, regions, organs, cells and processes of the organism toward life defines optimal health. To breathe is to live. To breathe fully is to thrive. To stop breathing signals death. This is true for the whole organism as well as each cellular component. It follows then that *to breathe with limitation limits the life force and the experience of living.* Unfortunately, for the vast majority of people, breathing habits are hindered by infinite variables, resulting in dissatisfaction, depression and disease. Nothing affects so negatively the sense of well-being and general state of health as does the habit of poor breathing. And no other vital function is so ignored.

Destiny of *The Pattern of The Breath*:
Differences in energetic capacities among individuals are reflected in *the breath.* More than any other distinct, defining dynamic of a personality is the constant, unique routine of *inhalation* and *exhalation* which absolutely determines the extent and quality of available energy. Again, this is a rational conclusion upheld by research and observation. How could it not be that those who breathe with fullness and smoothness over the course of a lifetime most assuredly must be healthier and less nervous and happier than those shallow breathers who seem never to relax? In fact, an astute trained observer can read the state of the inner world of a subject by noting the subtleties of posture, expression and, most telling, the *pattern of the breath.*

12

How you breathe is how you think, what you feel, what weaknesses you have and who you are. It is how you stand and what vibrations you send out to the world as well as your capacity to appreciate impressions you receive. No doubt, the quantity of fuel, its quality and efficiency of delivery establish how far, how fast, how long and how smoothly the organism can maneuver, adjust, avoid deterioration and possibly thrive. Over a lifetime, the ease and fullness of the way a person breathes mirrors the subjective measure of contentment.

Modern Progressive Medicine has just begun to realize that a person can learn to self-regulate physical reactions and emotional states through Breath-Work which can also revive natural healing energies. But this knowledge is in its infancy in the Western world, only studied on the fringes of the medical community. On the other hand, this is *age old* and *time worn* wisdom, practically employed by traditional cultures for thousands of years (often with cannabis). It accounts for the emphasis placed on breathing exercises in Yoga, Karate, Zen and other ancient but less-known indigenous disciplines.

Subtle Differences in Breathing Habits:
In complete contrast with Holistic Science, Modern Medicine does not recognize the *habit of the breath* as a measure of general health. In fact it is of no interest whatsoever! Only in the field of Psychiatry is severe breathing dysfunction linked to specific disorders. In some alternative schools of psychology, different states of mind are correlated to particular idiosyncrasies in breathing, such as contented mental states linked with deep inhalation and full exhalation, whereas nervousness is expressed in quick, shallow breathing. Panic attacks are known to accompany breathing dysfunction, triggered by a cognitive threat. But no treatment is offered by conventional doctors. No study exists in medical training concerning the extent that the *pattern of the breath* has on an individual profile of health.

Every emotion owns a unique breath pattern which is reflected in body chemistry and mirrored in mental field activity. Nothing is stagnant. Emotions are constantly changing synchronized with their corresponding way of breathing. Superior health is evidenced by appropriate changes in breathing as a reaction to any crisis at hand; once the crisis is over, the natural breath is easily and quickly resumed. In the holistic orientation, the time taken to return to normalcy is a measure of fitness. Should the crisis remain as a mental scar as is often the case, or if unpleasant, long-term situations are regularly feared, the breathing habit becomes understandably wounded, its functions weakened in kind. Health is equilibrium in emotions, balance of autonomic functions accompanied by deep and unrestricted breathing. The reverse is equally true. That is, deep and unrestricted breathing results in balance of autonomic process as well as steadiness in emotions, resulting in optimal (uncommon) vitality.

The Definition of *To Breathe*:

The Science of Breath is an ancient secret science. For the most part, it is hidden from the mainstream by virtue of its complexity as well as by the fact that little cultural value is lent to time for disciplined self-re-training when an aerosol *aid to breathing* is so easily obtained by doctor prescription. But esoteric knowledge is never lost. It is upheld by a living tradition that is continuously passed down by and for generation upon generation. It re-emerges from time to time when interest is re-stoked. The study of the breath can be a process of long-duration. For the most devoted students who delve into the profound cosmological meaning of "The Breath," it is actually a life-long pursuit.

In this very involved and complete science, the definition of *breathing* is not limited to inhalation and exhalation or the simple exchange of gases necessary to survive. It includes expansion and contraction of the thorax, motion of the chest, the abdomen, the interface of the organs, including nose, pharynx, larynx, trachea, bronchi and associative nerves and blood vessels. In addition, the individualized chemical responses to the specific mode of inspiration/expiration and the delicate energetic connection with mental processes are included in defining *the breath*. Breathing involves the whole being. Every cell breathes! And for every individual there is a different breathing rhythm that colors the physical, psychological and emotional experience.

The Routine of *The Breath*:
Throughout the day, there is an observable although nearly imperceptible alteration of nostril dominance that takes place. The regularity of the alteration has profound implications for self-development and ease of living. Nostril dominance is mirrored in brain process and therefore sets the stage for mood, intelligence and wellness. When the right nostril is flowing smoothly, the left brain hemisphere is most active, and the reverse is true. When the left nostril is flowing with ease, the right brain hemisphere is activated. Details of this knowledge with practical instructions to master them fill volumes in Eastern Science. Implications for health as well as evolution of consciousness are staggering.

Understanding that certain distortions in breathing rhythm are often linked to specific diseases is useful information that can be applied personally as well as in the professional capacity of Holistic Health Practitioner. The disease of Schizophrenia exhibits breathing with inordinate right nostril dominance often associated with left cerebral hemisphere dysfunction. The syndromes of Depression as well as The Cancer Biopathy are associated with excessive left-nostril dominance which is reflected in right brain overactive dysfunction.

When both sides of the brain are thoroughly integrated, the breath flows evenly from both nostrils. This rare state of pure equilibrium is defined as optimal health, evidenced in creativity, global thinking and compassion and experienced during a quiet mind.

The *Marijuana Breath:*

Administration of cannabis smoothes and regulates the daily alteration of nostril dominance simply because both brain hemispheres are innervated simultaneously in the Marijuana Effect. There is an energetic resonance that is variously described as awareness, peacefulness, liberation, bliss and any number of lofty adjectives. In addition, this state of equilibrium has been proven to activate the alpha state of brain relaxation. *The importance of this knowledge and how it pertains to healing is unknown in modern medicine. However, it has not been lost on the general population.* With the entry of Yoga Science into the West, coupled with the simultaneous influx of Marijuana into all levels of society, the ancient teachings of self discipline, personal growth and higher consciousness have been embraced from the grass roots upward.

Research into the Science of Marijuana has been a *grass-roots-driven* movement. Patients and activists together are responsible for exposing testimonials of thousands upon thousands of grateful medical Marijuana recipients. In addition, those citizens courageously demanded to be taken seriously which has made all the difference. Courage, determination and the truth overwhelmed the purposeful misinformation and the misplaced fear of the amazing medicinal plant.

16

Unflinching determination of those in the Marijuana movement despite the harsh laws of prohibition demonstrates the higher order of thinking that defines The Marijuana Consciousness wherein the intuitive dimension of human nature emerges. It seems fair to assume that the expanded consciousness has also served those who would/will not be silenced.

Chemical Imbalance IS Irregular Breathing*:*
Chemical imbalance is the contemporary *diagnosis-of-choice* for all mental unsteadiness, dissatisfaction and depression. It is considered an irreversible constitutional disease that is genetic. For the patient, this serves as comfort and actually encourages complete shirking of responsibility. No lifestyle change is considered. Daily habits are not examined. The Medical Model *Dogma of Faith* is set in place: *patient follows doctor's orders*. Small doses of lethal (expensive) drugs dampen the symptoms. As tolerance develops, stronger drugs are prescribed, with nary a momentary conjecture as to the origin of imbalance. D*rugs of Unconsciousness* lessen the gross symptom(s) through numbing expression of the disturbance while the on-going systemic sickness maintains. Its manifestation down the line is re-expressed in a seemingly unrelated and usually more severe disturbance, such as in the Cancer Biopathy.

*Marijuana Therapy***: Intuitive Remedy**:
The fact is that healthy breathing cannot exist in partnership to an unhealthy lifestyle. In fact, detrimental habits are but reflections of breathing dysfunction and its associative discomfort. Compensatory behaviors actually originate in and add to insufficient oxygenation. There is no mystery to the mechanical workings of the body or the mind. Just as when a carburetor does not mix its gases properly, the engine first sputters until it finally breaks down. No sane mechanic would suggest just drowning out the sputter with loud music. The carburetor must be reset.

In the same way, regardless what life insults have disturbed the smooth routine of the natural breath, once identified as the basic disturbance, suffice it to alter the problem in a practical, effective and time-worn way. Breath-Work, Meditation, Exercise and various Self Help-Disciplines are New Age Prescriptions for Health. Imagery, Amulets and Group-sharing are likewise in. But as we have noted: *The Benefits of Marijuana* are custom-tailored to both distortions and limitations in breathing which suggests that the incredibly large yet mostly illegal multi-billion dollar underground *Business of Marijuana* is an instinctive survival behavior of millions of citizens for all manifestation of imbalance borne of not having a full and relaxed *breath pattern*.

Marijuana is Not a Guarantee:
The Cancer Biopathy translates simply as an entity deprived of sufficient oxygen. Whatever can reverse that condition is needed. Marijuana increases oxygenation. It has myriad and varied benefits for hundreds of diseases (documented by Western research). In addition, marijuana patients testify to its relaxing and energizing effects, while the philosophy behind Holistic Health along with millennia-old wisdom hold that Marijuana Therapy is a *preventive and curative remedy for cancer.* Although surely not a guarantee, anyone who maintains a long-term regimen of Marijuana Therapy as a lifestyle diminishes the odds of developing cancer. (see Part III)

Presenting Symptom vs. Root Cause:
The underpinnings of Holistic Health and conventional medicine are philosophically opposed. The modern orientation considers the symptom itself to be the problem with no agenda to seek out where the illness originated. Chronic stomach problems are treated with antacids. *No sense examining the diet.* There is no *confidence* in a patient's ability to alter lifelong bad habits. In addition there are no practical *instructions* for how to accomplish such a drastic change.

The doctor has *no time* to search out the root cause. The patient just wants to feel better. Western Pharmacologic Medicine attacks the symptom, clear and simple. Any tumor (expression of imbalance) is cut out, poisoned, and burnt. In contrast, Holistic Health realizes that imbalance is at the core of illness. The goal is therefore to work toward restoring equilibrium. This can only be accomplished if the organism is not further destabilized via caustic treatments. The symptom is not considered the problem. It is a clue to the underlying distortion. The patient is co-detective with the Holistic Practitioner. Both take an active role in locating the problem and determining appropriate treatment.

A Cancerous Tumor is:
    Disordered Tissue that has become Toxic;
    An Intelligent *coping mechanism* to Limit
    The Contamination from Spreading.

The Body/Mind Link is *The Breath*:
Any tension in the breath displays in the body / mind field as a different facet of stress and negatively affects cellular chemistry. Noticing what happens to breathing and the body whenever there is any threat demonstrates the link between the body, the mind and *the breath*. Thought alone can trigger an adrenaline rush. The connection between the thought and the chemistry is none other than *the breath*. Fear is seen in inhibited breathing. A relaxed mind breathes with calm constancy and is experienced as comfort. It is a truism that is usually overlooked to state that a body at ease automatically has a regular free-flowing habit of the breath translated as mental calm. Expansion in the mind, of the breath, throughout all body systems and including all components of the cellular network is the natural, logical, visible and measurable result of full and deep breathing. The *Marijuana Breath* affords a deep sense of relief because of its unique action of relaxing and energizing at the same time which results in more oxygen and better delivery. (Benefits of Marijuana)

Chemical imbalance does not exist in an organism that breathes with full, slow, rhythmic and deep constancy. Increased brain integration occurs with marijuana* and is a direct result of more oxygen being accessible for cerebral activity. Sometimes expansion in *the breath* can be unsettling or it might even be uncomfortable. Sometimes it has psychological overtones. Nevertheless, after a short time, the *breathing-challenged-individual* accommodates to the higher energetic charge.

In the *World of Prescription Drugs*, overdose is the result of taking just a little more poison than the cells can stand or constricting breathing with anti-depressants, pain medications or chemotherapy just a little more than allows for living. The bottle may say dosage, but the connotation is danger and death. Take more than is ordered, and the results can be dire.

In *the World of The Marijuana Breath, a little more breathing than one is used to or a bit more fuel and nourishment than the cells habitually are allowed may be a tad disorienting until there is adjustment to the high octane fuel.*

The Marijuana Breath
Resets Body Chemistry
It Oxygenates.
It Nourishes.
It Dissolves the Cancer Biopathy.

(*documentation in The <u>Benefits of Marijuana</u>)

The Constant of the Breath Pattern:
The pattern of the breath is persistent and consistent. It is a lifetime constant from childhood. Only intentional, sustained intervention will alter the habit of 17,280 breaths taken every day by the normal person. It is stunningly clear that the continuous individualized habit of the breath shapes thoughts, behaviors and feelings. Health depends on how deeply one regularly breathes, how smooth is the intake, how efficient is the energy delivery and how full is the expiration. The successful organism functions as an integrated whole comprised of trillions of cells with billions of ongoing bio/chemical electro-magnetic interactions. The smoothest, steadiest and most enjoyable experience results from optimum fueling as a result of unimpeded breathing. Conversely, limitations in the amount, quality or delivery of energy define an organism that may survive but cannot flourish since thoughts, emotions and perceptions are degraded. While a person may endure into longevity, subtleties in the breathing pattern make all the difference as to how those many years are spent.

Accompaniments to the Healthy Breath:
Nourishment: Holistic Health views personal lifestyle as a mirror of the individual *pattern of the breath*. Habits, preferences, values and perceptions, even interpretations are understood as outgrowths of the specific level of one's energetic vitality. It follows that the continuous routine of the energizing breath serves as the foundation for each unique life experience which in turn sets the style of life. The emphasis on *The Breath* in traditional Wisdom is not an exercise in knowledge. Very simply: all things are colored by the way that we breathe. While it is nearly impossible to change thinking patterns and/or to alter mechanical behaviors borne from specific breathing deficits, to enhance the breath can be accomplished with intention and attention. (Breathing is volitional **or** automatic: the feature that allows it to be altered. (a vast topic – not covered in this presentation.)

The natural breath results in an organism drawn to appropriate choices, such as: eating, relating and thinking because balance and security exist at the cellular level. While breath is the primary nourisher of life, of course what is digested by the body and what vibrational impressions are ingested into the psyche contribute to the subject's overall state of being. Not relaxed; eat on the go; not digesting correctly; not sufficient elimination indicate anxiety, tension and fear and in no way describe what is implied by the *healthy breath*. Poor breathing creates poor habits which destabilize yet further the automatic internal processes. Marijuana Therapy automatically restores stability. Peristalsis increases. Taste is heightened. The individual is relaxed. Elimination is expedited resulting in toxins being moved out of the body quicker; and Marijuana raises blood velocity, serving rapid efficient filtration.

Balance: Balance of the organism by way of Marijuana Therapy is accomplished through oppositional modes of action. If there is lethargy, movement is toward stimulation, so that the effect changes along with the state of the subject. Relaxation is generally associated with marijuana, simply because modern life is so fast-paced. There is a skewing toward over-stimulation. For healthy balance, our systems usually need to be **toned down** *and chilled out*. Balance defines an organism whose internal, automatic activities, such as, respiration; blood pressure; digestion; circulation, etc. reflect flexibility to challenge. Inhibited Breathing, on the other hand produces chronic and rigid imbalance, experienced as dis-ease, evidenced in mood swings, nervousness and dissatisfaction. It is a chronic *state of (suffocated) being, known as the stress that kills.*

The circular effect in the pattern of the breath is that tension results from repressed breathing while repressed breathing causes tension. Practical wisdom garnered from Ancient Traditions teaches to intervene directly at the source. The feature with the greatest potential for restoration of equilibrium is undoubtedly *the breath*. Western Medicine prescribes tranquilizers which further and foolishly depress *the breath* and consequently the energy, its delivery and quality so that the patient doesn't feel better, just less. On the contrary, Marijuana Therapy enlivens the process of breathing while increasing the efficacy of its flow as well as its delivery throughout the relaxed and receptive organism. Therefore, **the person feels better and more!**

Security: The Ending of Insecurity:
The *holistic* understanding is an inclusive philosophy where there really is no separation between body and mind. Logically speaking, if there is lacking in the fuel at the cellular level, subjective sensing and registration (*feelings*) of insecurity at the psychological level automatically will reflect that insufficient oxygenation. To feel safe and to relax, survival must be assured for the whole person as a unified incorporation of energy. As a personality feature, insecurity manifests as a state of generalized anxiety referenced in psychiatric jargon as *Generalized Anxiety Disorder* (GAD), appropriately described as frozen fear.

In fact, anxiety as a way of being is a long-standing unconscious and defective coping mechanism that is carried out by inhibiting the breath. *The Natural Breath* and Insecurity are at opposing ends of the continuum of health. A sense of well-being or as the IOM put it: a *good mood consciousness* is produced with Marijuana Therapy - accompanied by deep and regular respiration.

Dis-ease: Imbalance/Cause/Prevalence

Dysfunctional Circle of Chronic Illness:
Chronic illness (*Disease*) follows from an individual coping with being deprived of what he or she needs over a long period of time. First and foremost, of course is sufficient oxygenation, without which there is lasting imbalance that becomes- unfortunately - comfortably familiar but necessarily encourages compensatory damaging behaviors. Poor nutrition and eating habits, excessive stimulation, negative thinking and any number of long-term habits, settings, and even relationships can further degrade the energetic flow which leaves less awareness for health.

In the child developmental stage, insufficient emotional support or ongoing intimidation or worse predictably results in restricted breathing as a habitual way to ward off sadness and deaden feelings. It is carried through the adult life imprinted with stress. It is systemic imbalance and whole person uneasiness played out in over-active adrenals, excess cortisol, retained CO_2, diminished circulation, etc., oftentimes devolving to chaos at the cellular level and/or confusion in the mind, thereby diagnosed as the popular fad of *chemical imbalance*.

Stress can likewise be viewed as habitual incompetency in meeting challenge which reflects the consistent personality disequilibrium that is an automatic bio-chemical response to anything perceived as threatening. Stress is reflected in types of thinking, ways of feeling, behaving and accompanied always by insufficiency in the *pattern of the breath*. Rather than a relaxed personality, stress tells of tension that is almost an ingrained personality feature that is circular in nature with accompanying behaviors that are instantaneously triggered and are not easily altered. The whole being is upset which after long duration often results in one of the *named diseases* depending upon the individual constitutional weakness.

24

Remediation for Stress according to Holistic Health is to reinstate the gentle vibration of easy breathing which immediately dissolves all accompanying problems and allows the organism to maintain equilibrium in the face of life. Everyone is unique and reacts differently. External circumstances cannot be controlled. But reactions can be checked. The goal for health and healing is to stop the *stress response* from becoming exaggerated and chronic. It needs to be **toned down.** Marijuana Therapy restores the autonomic regulatory mechanism of the organism. It *Moderates, Modulates and Regulates the functioning of the human organism* and **tones down** over-reactivity.

Common Breathing Dysfunction: Who Can Breathe*?* Since almost all adults do not breathe fully, nor have they over the course of years, their lung capacity diminishes with age. *What is not used is lost.* Without healthy diaphragmatic breathing, there is less oxygen for consumption. Less is distributed. Less gaseous waste is expelled and more is retained. Blood velocity slows resulting in less filtration (*tired blood*). Without a continuous, conscious attempt to stem the destruction of the *tide of time*, less and less efficient and sufficient breathing occurs with each passing year.

Adults average lung capacity could be 6 liters of air (approx. volume), but the average adult takes in only ½ liter per breath. This depressing statistic is the result of (perceived) long-standing emotional abuse. Human beings cope with fear, pain and anger by diminishing the intake and outgo of the breath. It is an instinctive, but ill-advised maneuver. Less breathing translates to less feeling. Everyone has developed unique, life-long breath patterns in response to experience. As children, chronic disapproval easily manifests as loss of full breathing. As the society becomes more competitive, there is ever more tension and less breath.

With the ever increasing atmospheric pollution, chronic breathing dysfunction escalates resulting in increased childhood asthma, COPD and Cancer.

The older we get, the more restricted breathing becomes. Toxins that should/could be exhaled instead become stuck in the cells. Clogged arteries create further degradation. Obesity, poor nutrition and worry just exacerbate further the already diminished breath. For most adults, breathing is far removed from the effortless inhalation and exhalation of an infant and/or a still carefree/healthy child. Over time, imperceptible but constant lack of suitable oxygenation degrades into insufficient immune response and subsequent increase in inflammation. At the later stage of accumulated cellular under-aeration, materialization of cellular suffocation is diagnosed as cancer.

Disturbed Breathing and Specific Diseases:
Although no such information is readily available, in fact, the subtle, barely noticed nuances of depth, speed, rhythm and smoothness of the habitual breathing practice are inherently tied to the personal sense of well-being and the actual wellness of the organism. The chest breather is known to be anxiety prone, paradoxical breathing habits are associated with schizophrenia, insufficient expiration is the signature of asthma, ADD can be traced to inhaling before fully exhaling, cardiac problems are accompanied by pauses in breathing *(apnea)*. The list of illnesses associated with specific dysfunction in the breath is very extensive and well documented in Holistic Health, yet hardly mentioned in conventional medical education: certainly, it is a non-entity for the lay population, such as the cancer patient.

The way an individual breathes expresses and causes the emotional constitution. By the same logic which recognizes the circular effects of breathing, it is clear that emotional content of the personality is absolutely extended to the breathing pattern, which then upholds the emotional profile. Fright causes breath-holding, sadness is seen in jerks in the breath while relief is denoted by a sigh. Repetitive situations that cause fright, despair or other negativity are projected into the future as chronic restricted patterns in the breath. By the same logic, emotional content is absolutely extended to the breathing pattern.

Marijuana has its Most Noticeable Fundamental Benefit at the Level of *The Breath.*

Cancer is Oxygen Depletion

Consequences of Limitation in Breathing:
When breathing is chronically constrained in any fashion from any cause, specific areas or regions of the organism are deprived of adequate sustenance. It may take years for the enduring deprivation to develop into an illness. It may be that the chronic limitation in breathing presents primarily as mental imbalance. Regardless how an illness is classified, its origin was a disruption in the breath. The subtleties of the distinctive way a person breathes are as numerous as there are people. Almost everyone has some wound that has created a glitch in the perfect breath pattern.

Cancer Evolves from Restricted Breath:
Cancer is linked to the subdued and shallow breath which denotes fearfulness and quiet resignation. *Shallow Breathing of the Chest Breather* causes the *alarm reaction* by stimulating the Sympathetic Nervous System and is associated with the chemicals that help the organism to flee in the face of danger or to fight. It is a threefold action: *become activated; deal with the danger; recover from the activity.* In modern times, however, the alarm is activated habitually, unnecessarily via the mental interpretation of threats to the ego, the pocketbook or the imagined future. There are no lions lurking around the corner. There is, however, a constant feeling of having to achieve with its accompanying worry of how one will perform. A person who is on guard or on the go, most of the time describes the habitual chest breather, notorious for low immune resistance because of disregarded exhaustion. There is rarely the deep, relaxed and rhythmic breathing (diaphragmatic) needed to innervate the Parasympathetic Nervous System which allows for relaxation. *Subdued breathing* signifies resignation from long standing or overwhelming sadness. It suggests a loss of thrust toward the survival intent owing to decreased energy.

In combination with the shallow breath which keeps the organism charged via body chemicals, the subdued habit of the breathing mechanism creates a non-rhythmic pattern and an intermittent delivery of energy to the cells. Repressing emotions over painful experiences is seen in the quiet, subdued and very shallow breathing which is a harbinger of future disease. In the cancer-prone individual, feelings of helplessness are hidden by suppressing the breath. Less breathing is equivalent to feeling less. Inhibited breath deprives not only the emotions but also the trillions of cells that comprise the whole. Systemic Imbalance is the result.

Total volume of air that the lungs can contain is termed *Vital Capacity*. A more apt term cannot be imagined.

28

Holistic Explanation of Cancer:
The healthy organism is the sum of billions of cells working in concert out from which a synchronous vibration emanates. There really is no difference between the body, the mind or the energetic components of an individual life. The notion that cancer comes from the mind refers to a breakdown in the operation of the whole entity that was first foretold in a vibration of imbalance which over time made itself visible (i.e., became manifest) on the concrete plane. The breath fuels the immeasurable interconnections among all elements of the organism. Each cell lives and breathes as a working component of the whole but also as a contained entity on its own. When oxygenation is chronically insufficient to an area, stagnation is the outcome. There is lack of aeration, poor filtration, failed communication, loss of cooperation among cells and finally degradation. Regardless of the obstacle that limits the breath; *undernourished cells separate from the whole that has betrayed them.* The neglected areas attempt to survive in whatever way is feasible. Cancer is born of suffocation. Cancer is fermentation.

Cancer is Adaptation of Suffocated Cells.
Acting as Self-Sustaining Units
No Longer Committed to the Whole.
It Failed to Nourish Them. It Did Not Protect Them.
Neither Did It Maintain Balance.
They are Striking Out (on their own)
Without the Luxury of Oxygen.

Survival is the Goal:

Cancer is essentially a survival tactic wherein the higher order of cooperative co-existence in an oxygen rich environment has been lost to the cellular template and a more primal technique for survival has been adopted as necessity. To survive, the suffocating cells disconnect from the whole. They take on a life of their own and adopt the primitive form of energizing themselves. They begin an anaerobic life (living without oxygen) of fermentation (rotting)! Cancer cells do not use oxygen. Instead, by having been deprived of needed oxygen, they instinctively revert back to the anaerobic pattern of growing and dividing independently without responding to the usual regulation of the body. They give up and leave usual metabolic pathways that were insufficient to maintain the sophistication of oxygenated life. That is, there simply was not enough oxygen for the entire organism. The result is cancer in some system or organ.

Personality Signature of Cancer: (TYPE C)

The weakness that often portends the **Cancer Biopathy** can be measured by means of the distribution of energy throughout the organism and consequential displays of *areas of unconsciousness. The Type C personality* often demonstrates a tendency to disregard unpleasant realities by denial and repression of accompanying emotions, accomplished by also suppressing the breath. The coping style of a Type C personality may be seen in depression as a way to not face problems or may be couched in extreme busy work to deny feelings of helplessness. Regardless of the external presentation, repressed emotions represent expressions of energetic disturbance which will sooner or later, manifest as an area of neglect. Negativity does not allow for full and complete exhalation, which is stasis at the cellular level. Research points to loss in Immune System competency in reaction to psychological stress. The translation of mental disturbance to a physical disease takes place via distortion in breathing.

Psychologically Speaking:

The *tendency toward cancer* of a particular personality type is served by a characterological tension. Basically, from a simplified point of view, it can be said that the emotions are held in check – chronically! The constraint is accomplished via shallow breathing almost all of the time. Marijuana allows for a deep relaxation of the entire psyche. The up-tight, on-guard, striving, worrying and overly busy mode which is directly responsible for so many types of modern chronic disease gives way to a less invested, more accepting, less needy and fearful orientation which is not fertile ground for the seeds of the Cancer Syndrome. Relaxation can be equated to improvement in the gaseous exchange (breathing) in all the cells of the body from *the Marijuana Effect*. This allows for a higher functionality in the nervous system including the integrative processes of the brain so often visible in creative expression; and so often lost with the dread diagnosis of cancer.

The benefits of marijuana are not limited to the physicality of the full breath. With cancer patients who employ Marijuana Therapy, the extension outward toward creativity can serve as forward-looking and naturally healing borne of the diminished worry/tension that accompanies deep aeration of the entire being. It is relevant to note that recent research has proven that marijuana promotes the development of new cells in the hippocampus region of the brain, thereby reducing anxiety and depression!!

(The topic is too extensive to cover in this presentation.)

The Constricted Breath of the Cancer Biopathy
Immediately Released by The Marijuana Effect

When The Immune System is Compromised:
Chronic deprivation becomes inflammation at the cellular level, psychologically analogous to *stress or inflamed emotional reactivity* which unfortunately describes a common-place entrenched way of breathing and being. Many tranquilizing drugs are prescribed for this particular distress which serves to mask the underlying problem. But without rehabilitating the imbalanced lifestyle, the Immune System becomes weakened. It cannot ward off the consequences of inflammation, stagnation and putrification.

Long term suffocation, a result of continuous diminished breathing, is a whole person experience and expression wherein accesses to finer, healing energies are inaccessible. (Part III). Suffice it to point out that once the Cancer Biopathy is visibly manifest, survival has already progressed to a frantic alienated *celf-centered* endeavor. The Immune Response is dysfunctional. Systemic cooperation is lost as cells can be said to become selfish since they are outside the goal of holistic synchrony for the benefit of the whole. Alienation and lack of communication are in charge of the operation.

When the whole organism is working as an integrated composite, the prime directive is survival! The Immune Response transports, dissolves and disintegrates necrotic and contaminating cells to disposal outside the body. But with dysregulation of the Immune Response, what happens is non-directed development and spreading of chaotic growth.

The Energetic Deficiency that is the Natural Consequence of Partial Suffocation is Immediately Replenished by the Marijuana Effect.

Loss of Balance in All Human Endeavors:

True Healing takes place when/if the human organism can maintain equilibrium within the context of the chaos of modern life. At every turn situations are present that invite imbalance:

- The Food - Deficiencies in the soil borne from the glut of toxic fertilizers degrade food sources and poison the waters. Modern diets are contaminated with hormones, animal fat, genetically-altered veggies, concentrated sugars and excessive salts, all of which spell predictable sickness in the collective society;

- The Air - Atmospheric pollution drastically limits oxygen which affects not only the physical body but the caliber of thinking;

- The Culture - Excess stimulation as a lifestyle sets the stage for a concurrent need for depressants: alcohol and tranquilizers;

Understandably, most humans are suffering from **gross imbalance** evidenced in large-scale immunological insufficiency; increasing cases of chronic inflammatory disturbances, pervasive nutritional deficiencies in conjunction with obesity along with inordinate feelings of confusion and dismay among a large cross section of the population, especially the younger generations. This assortment of maladies is a definite pre-cursor to the Cancer Biopathy and upholds the unfortunate reality that Cancer is on the rise.

Cancer was the third leading cause of death in the wealthiest countries for years but will soon be #1; more than 12 million deaths annually will be from cancer in the next decade. The shameful statistic from the World Health Organization is that 40% of cancer deaths are preventable and that altering the individual lifestyle is the way to avoid disease. Truth is: unless the breath is released, the addiction to alcohol, tobacco and poor diet too often cannot be overcome.

There is no longer any doubt that Marijuana is the herb of choice to raise awareness, to release tensions of normal living, to balance the body/mind and thereby raise the quality of life, while simultaneously affording the person the strength in conscious intent to alter whatever is a detrimental habit. But for the collective society to avail itself of the vast *benefits of marijuana*, a complete about-face in values is needed. Self responsibility for one's own health is far different from the encouraged passivity of today's medical model. Ironically, most cancer deaths occur under Medical Care where the treatments are ultimately so energetically debilitating and unbearable that the organism dies. The *prime directive of causing no harm* is lost in the battle against the *enemy* named cancer, while the main goal to help the person to rebalance is forgotten. Tobacco, obesity and alcohol rank as the top three causes of cancer by modern measure. In actual fact, the root cause can be traced back to a suffocating organism that is seeking solace in all the wrong places.

The Automatic Progression of the Cancer Syndrome Can Be Completely Reversed by The Holistic Therapy of Marijuana

Note: The root of *anxiety* (defined herein as prolonged stress) is *to strangle*, implying that the correlation between long-term insufficient breathing (which causes anxiety) was known many years ago.

PART II

The Cannabinoid System

Compatibility with Marijuana:

Marijuana Therapy is a very specific and complex encountering that occurs between the body and the components of Cannabis that has only recently been defined and appreciated from the standpoint of biology. The medical, recreational and religious history of the plant can be traced back thousands of years, but only in the last few generations has its molecular composition become known. Research has discovered an ancient, essential and beneficial relationship between the compounds of cannabis and human physiology. Vast numbers of scientific projects have been and are being devoted to the study of Marijuana and its promise for health. Almost all of these studies are conducted outside U.S. borders because of the reigning philosophy of prohibition. But the results cannot be repressed.

The discovery of what has aptly been named **The Cannabinoid System** in the human body was surely the scientific find of the past century. How such a basic and pervasive biochemical cellular mechanism escaped notice is proof positive of the fallibility of objective science. In fact, discovery of this intricate structural set of connections was accidental, uncovered only as a consequence of research on Marijuana. Yet in less than a decade, this sophisticated **Signaling System** has been acknowledged as the *basic regulating cellular network of all earth-organisms (not insects).*

The Cannabinoid System can be traced backward in time some 500 plus million years to well before the emergence of homo-sapiens. It actually pre-dates the evolution of land animals, making its entrance on the scene of planetary creatures in the simple and very ancient mollusk. No doubt, the evolution of its balancing function has played a crucial role in shaping whatever species that has followed

Throughout the evolutionary progression, the efficiency of The Cannabinoid System has been scrupulously conserved. Its development that the human and the clam both share is clouded by hundreds of millions of years not-yet-translated by the technology of this century.

What Science has Documented:
The complex, numerous and unique compounds of Cannabis Sativa evolved hundreds of millions of years ago, although vagueness concerning the evolution and appearance on the planet still surrounds seed bearing plants... *intractable a mystery today as it was to Darwin 130 years ago.* (Rothwell *et al.* 2009) As far back as there are records, Cannabis Sativa and human society have been intertwined. It was not a chance happening that drew ancient cultures to Marijuana but instead, what can now be understood as, an inherent *biological magnetism* to its effects. Between the compounds of Cannabis and the human organism, there is a genetic compatibility that has been proven beyond a shadow of a doubt validating the intuitive wisdom of the oldest societies by science.

Humans were obviously drawn to Marijuana for its multitude of uses and pleasures. It is less clear why a particular plant would be so persistently a companion to humans. An oft offered hypothesis is that the seeds quite naturally self-planted themselves and thrived in the disturbed soils of early settlements. Other more mystical theories have even suggested that the plant surmised human involvement would further its own survival. Whatever may be the details of the past, the ancient Cannabis Sativa plant and human development are termed "co-evolutionary" by historians.

Marijuana Compounds: (*Cannabinoids*)
There are Three Classifications of Cannabinoids:
1) Chemical compounds of Cannabis Sativa;
2) Chemical compounds of Earth creatures; and
3) Chemical compounds synthesized in the Lab.

There are approximately 500 compounds that make-up Marijuana. Only 60 are considered active by the scientist although t*hat number has recently risen to 80.* These are the oil based, aromatic and thoroughly unique molecules found in abundance in the fruit of Cannabis Sativa and fittingly named cannabinoids. Very recently, nine hitherto unknown cannabinoids have been found:

> *Two are of the cannabichromene type (CBC), one is the cannabigerol type (CBG) and the other two are classified with the cannabinols (CBNs) known to have significant antibacterial activities. (J. Nat. Prod.)*

This quote just hints at the complex interactions that must occur in a mix of more than 80 *active* molecules and some 400 or so that have been disregarded as inactive, suggesting they are unimportant.

> *It is not merely the monopoly of drug companies that causes concern. Many are worried about the dangers of isolating so-called active ingredients. One danger is that the modifying agents are left out. Modifying agents are the part of the make-up of some herbs which render the whole herb safe. These may not appear 'active' in isolated tests, but they offset the side effects of the active constituents.* Lesley Bremness: <u>World of Herbs</u>

Discovery of The Cannabinoids:

THC is famous for its *high. It was the first cannabinoid discovered.* Now, just a few decades later, seventy-nine additional cannabinoids have been found in Marijuana and many of them are emerging as *stars in their own right by demonstrating p*owerful healing abilities for the human organism that are astounding the researchers.

Cannabinoids produced by Marijuana are known as *exogenous* because they are *exterior* to the body. Over the last few decades, there has been stringent science proving that *Flower cannabinoids, (phyto-chemicals) of Cannabis Sativa, have a momentous balancing effect on human physiology, experienced as relief from tension.* (Marijuana: *Reliever of Distress* in ancient India')

Not long after THC was discovered, its interactive processes with the human organism were traced. Scientific consensus pointed to the likelihood that THC wielded its effects by fitting receptors that were designed for similar chemicals actually made by the body. **En**dogenous Cannabinoids are produced inside the Body. Mechoulam (et al) discovered *Anandamide,* which ended the search for the **body chemical** with marijuana-type effects. The **endo**genous, oil-based cannabinoid was fittingly named Ananda (*Bliss* in Sanskrt) to honor *The Marijuana Experience.* Up until that time, the mechanism by which the natural molecules impact its own body had not yet been located. Originally what was exposed by the discovery of Anandamide was unclear. It pointed to the molecules of Marijuana and also its endogenous counterpart as innervating a *major* (neurotransmission) system of the organism that was not even known to exist. In fact, it appeared that the phyto-chemicals of the Plant were (are) actually a functioning **Master Key** that unlocks a cascade of physiological, extremely refined equalizing effects through cellular relay stations that were never seen or even imagined

The CB1 Receptor:

Ongoing research has established that there are specific cellular receivers that are activated by both THC and *Anandamide*. The first receiver to be found is now well-known as the CB1 Receptor. With the avalanche of research and knowledge that is ongoing, other body messenger molecules have been located that activate yet other recently discovered Receptors. The Receptors, the body messenger endogenous cannabinoids, including the interactive processes by which they affect the organism comprise The Cannabinoid System.

Plant cannabinoids and endogenous cannabinoids are different in shape, length of life and duration of action. But their message is transmitted via the same sophisticated and subtle electro-magnetic operation. Surprisingly, studies show that the Cannabinoid Receptors demonstrate a greater affinity for Sativa cannabinoids than for those of its own body, which may suggest some type of primal recognition.

What is known at this time is that there is much still not known. Many yet-to-be found body cannabinoids surely exist; some may even have their effects without linking up to Cannabinoid Receptors; many probably imitate the interrelated effects of one or more of the known plant cannabinoids. The obvious synergy among Endogenous Cannabinoids, along with their beneficial interactions with the Exogenous compounds is consistently and historically resisted by conventional science.

Consensus among the established scientific community is that yet more proof is needed. It will assuredly be forthcoming. It will, furthermore, clearly reveal the complicated and quite instantaneous interconnections among body and plant cannabinoids and the all pervasive Cannabinoid Network that serves to re-balance the destabilized system.

Brilliant Cannabinoid System

Transmitters and Receivers:
Within the living organism, there is a cellular dynamism and communication that is constant. There are trillions of multi-faceted and constantly replicating cells that comprise the body. Nothing is static. Every cell is interacting with its internal and external environment on a nano second-to-second basis with a multitude of operations, orchestrated through and by components of (unknown) specificity. Communication within the body occurs through **cellular messaging stations** which receive, interpret and forward chemical/electrical and even magnetic signals for the supremely complex communication of all systems, such as the Nervous System, Circulatory System, Digestive System, etc. Directing all these processes is the network of receivers and transmissions: The Cannabinoid System.

The language of body messaging is particularized by function. That is, different chemicals secreted by the **transmitter** part of a cell serve as instructions to another part of another cell with special receptors to decipher the message. The Receptor's shape, location and derivative determine if it will accept and/or can follow instructions of the transmission. Receptors can be likened to the key hole of a lock. The key that fits the lock activates the process. In the case of the living entity, when the right molecule (the transmission) comes floating by in the matrix between the cells, the Receptor engages. Cells have different kinds and quantities of these microscopic locks sometimes numbering in the hundreds. There are just as many message-molecules floating around to inform the cells what to do at any given moment.

Myriad Functions of Cannabinoids:

The Cannabinoid System is everywhere in the body. Its receptors are dispersed throughout organs, systems and just about all cells. It serves essential homeostatic functions which allow for life to begin and to continue. For the past **500 million years**, all vertebrate species have utilized CB1 Receptors, found in most tissue, even skin, while CB2 Receptors are mostly in the Immune System. There are other Cannabinoid Receptors - recent evidence pointing to one connected to pain.

Even with so much more to learn, it is known that **The Cannabinoid System is the Largest Neurotransmitter Network of the Brain and Immune System** comprised of Receptors, *Messaging Molecules* and its myriad processes. This primary coordinating system is super-attuned to the *Cannabinoids of the Sativa*. The Cannabinoid System is a network of hundreds of millions (perhaps billions) of relay stations throughout the body that serve as a *balancing association* that is *always engaged but inconspicuous* in operation.

When the Cannabinoid Network is debilitated, balance is off, stress is high and the all-system disturbance is prelude to illness. Cannabinoid Receptors operate independently, locally and in sync with the Maintainer of Harmony (Hypothalamus of the Brain) of automatic bodily processes (BP, HR, Temperature, etc.). Rather than initiating cellular activity, The Cannabinoid System operates through complex, interdependent cross-communicative flux of information to *tone down* excess. It works in its homeostatic function with an immediacy that appears intuitive and is reflected and experienced in mental well-being. That *High-Feeling,* denounced as a disadvantage by the Pharmaceutical giants is nothing but childlike and, unfortunately lost subjective experience of an optimally functioning Cannabinoid System.

Scientists report that the brain produces proteins that act like marijuana...this) may lead to **new marijuana-like drugs** for pain, appetite and **preventing marijuana abuse ... and** will lead to drugs that bind to and activate the THC Receptor, but are *devoid of the side effects that limit usefulness of marijuana.* (Science Daily, 2009)

The Endo Cannabinoid System works as an understated behind-the-scenes Manager-Monitor of the automatic processes of balancing, moderating and modulating extreme reactions. Cannabinoids are only synthesized when needed for any number of the complex regulatory actions of the network. There is an ever-present, multi-tasking communication that takes place at the cellular level and operates via an uncommon manner of chemical signaling (known in scientific jargon as "retrograde messaging). Between the physiology of the human being and the Marijuana compounds, there is a stunning enthusiastic molecular compatibility which is fundamental to **How Marijuana Cures Cancer.**

The Cannabinoid System: Disease / Dysfunction:
The impact of The Cannabinoid System on the quality of life is dramatic! The list of its fundamental directives grows every week. It is essential to survival throughout the entire life-cycle for every Earth creature. Dysfunction in the Cannabinoid System portends disharmony and disease and in progressive scientific circles, a deficient Cannabinoid System IS a *disease (EDCS).* (**http://www.alternet.org/story/146151/**

> *Scientists speculating on the **cause of disease have determined ... that Endo-Cannabinoid Deficiency Syndrome is a basic malfunction** Endo-cannabinoids (and their interaction with Cannabinoid Receptors... throughout the body) play a key role in regulation of proper appetite, anxiety control, blood pressure, bone mass, reproduction, motor coordination and more. (March 24, 2010) (*ECD)*

What happens when the body cannot produce enough cannabinoids? *'It's called 'Cannabinoid Deficiency.'* (Al Byrne of Patients Out of Time). Could craving for cannabinoids be a symptom of **Cannabinoid Deficiency Syndrome**? *'Certainly patients who have a wasting disease are cannabinoid deficient, which might explain why these patients are helped by ingesting marijuana.'*

Restoration of Cannabinoid System:
Although so far, only a limited number of researchers have stepped onto the ledge of truth, nevertheless, the knowledge that insufficiency of the Cannabinoid System is directly correlated with the development of specific medical problems is quietly seeping and sometimes leaping into respectable scientific circles spurred on by the broadminded curiosity of young scientists. In the more conventional circles, a great deal of caution prevails for two reasons: (1) New and innovative science is naturally difficult to swallow for entrenched professionals; and *more to the point: (2) The remedy for a defunct Cannabinoid System is Marijuana*!

There is no denying it. The Cannabinoid System directs the vital functions of life; responds to the phyto-cannabinoids of the ancient Cannabis Sativa plant with a kind of prehistoric recognition! Generally, it appears if the Cannabinoid Network does not function optimally, imbalance, diminished ability to cope, and disease result. The imbalance is noticeably and quickly relieved with Marijuana Therapy. The organism recuperates, regains strength and disease dissolves.

NB: The previous theoretical explanation represents a better-than *best case scenario*. In real life, all kinds of contingencies can cause mental and physical confusion and suffering. Who will employ Marijuana Therapy as a prime treatment if the diagnosis is life-threatening? Especially with the entire medical philosophy and community in opposition to natural treatment, how many can withstand the pressure?

In the case of the Cancer Syndrome: time is needed for reversal of entrenched cellular distortion as an accompaniment to diminished breathing. The patient may not have enough time or at least may be warned that time is short and not following modern treatments will have dire results. Chemotherapy, radiation and/or surgery will be prescribed. What is clear, regardless of theory or prognostication, there is immediate *relief from distress* with Marijuana. Of course, dissolution of the tumour also takes time. There is always concern that the tumour has become too much of a challenge and may not diminish quickly enough. This may surrender the patient to the doctors who do not understand the gentle yet definite benefits of Marijuana. There are so many testimonials concerning the unmitigated recovery of terminal cancer patients on the internet whose tumours decreased very rapidly with Marijuana Therapy where modern medicine failed. Hopefully, soon, popular proof will filter upward to the Medical mindset so that unbiased science is conducted. Time is needed to repair tissue; for recuperation; and for changing destructive habits that may thwart healing. Regardless of the above mentioned obstacles for recovery from The Cancer Biopathy: **Marijuana Therapy is always indicated.**

Side Note:
The list of illnesses caused by ECDS is short since so little research has been done. AND there is hesitancy in admitting that the maligned Marijuana compounds are proving to be miraculous! Migraine relief was the first documented proof of the wonder of Marijuana Therapy since the disease was considered incurable. Marijuana Therapy renders the symptoms gone! On a personal note, *forty years of Marijuana Therapy has eliminated all signs of the disease.* Testimonials for the favourable effects of Marijuana on migraines were a major motivation for research in the early years. Today, patient testimony and evidence concerning the benefits of Marijuana for cancer are yet more compelling and the political and intellectual climate is far more hopeful.

Retrograde Operation of the Message

The Cannabinoid System Calms that which Excites.
It Excites that which Calms, Indirectly and Backwards!

Cannabinoid System: (Subtle, Dynamic Balance)
There is mystery in the mechanism of the Human
Cannabinoid System that cannot be fully incorporated
into the objective understanding of science. It can be
called _prior knowledge_ or _Retrograde Signaling_ or
Anticipatory Action. By whatever name, the uncommon
manner of signaling of The Cannabinoid System is one
of the reasons that it went undetected for so long. Its
unique and complicated style of signal transduction has
what is called "retrograde transmission," or reversed
flow of instruction. It doesn't just travel in the one-way
direction that is usual for transmitters and receivers.
That is, an instructional message to a cell typically
follows a forward course. Information goes to the
receiver from the transmitter (part of the cell) which is
actually why one part of the cell is given the name of
Receptor and another part of the cell is the Transmitter.
Retrograde Signaling, however, is not limited by the
straight and narrow program. Instead, the receiver may
actually be the transmitter and the transmitter may be the
receiver. And very often, this is a both/and operation.
From the Receiver certain information leaks and seeps
back to the Transmitter (through the fluid matrix
between cells) with a message that may inhibit that
which was about to be transmitted. Or it may not. It all
depends on how much and how often there is backward
seepage which depends on how much is anticipated as
needed for future balance (all taking place within and
without the cells via various regulating chemical
patterns.) This is a prescient recognition of what is
needed before the need is expressed. (Not sending
instruction can either allow or stop a future cellular
transmission.) Indeed, the receiver is actually controlling
its own messages.

Within this essential system, there is an intelligence that is constant in its vigilance **to tone down** all over-reactions which is termed Depolarization-induced Suppression of Inhibition (DSI). The opposite mode of The Cannabinoid System exhibits Depolarized-Induced Suppression of Excitation, known as DSE.

Retrograde signaling may not be exactly exclusive to cannabinoids. The literature suggests that different neuro-transmitters (there are many) might also be retrograde in some situations (or not). The evidence is not clear and the interpretations are murky, at best. With **cannabinoids**, however, *it is a sure thing*. The super-sophistication of its operation can be likened to anticipating what must be done (which includes doing nothing) to maintain balance nano-seconds before the challenge. Balance in flux is the Modus Operandi. In actuality, this process has many more steps which are simplified for logical, common-place comprehension. Nevertheless, the dual action of the Cannabinoid System, within its almost limitless boundaries of intra-cellular continuous processes, has the net effect of maintaining equilibrium of the organism always.

It Gives Pause
Over-Reactive Processes are Calmed

Body/Mind Interface:
Retrograde Signaling is a discovery worth far more than its biology. It is a momentary suspension in cellular activity, built into the homeostatic process and reflected in a corresponding hiatus from superficial chatter. It is experienced as relief / relaxation / well-being. Without constant underlying disharmony, finer energies (hitherto blocked by dissonance) can flow with ease. In fact, the suspension in thought is likened to the peaceful mind of esoteric disciplines. *No thought* is where opposites are magically merged since thinking is inherently dualistic and holds opposing opinions for all situations.

Either this *or* that is the continuous litany of trivialities of the mind, whereas with the ending of thought (or the pause in signal transduction which gives rise to an intermission in stimulation), i.e., dualism dissolves into unity referred to as *beyond the mind and cognitively registered as an alteration to a higher consciousness.*

Ergo: When the Cannabinoid System is in peak performance, the entire organism exudes ease, evident in the cells, in the breath and in the mind. The Cancer Biopathy stands exactly opposite to psychological calm and physical relaxation that is the signpost of health. The Br*eath of Resignation* characterizes Cancer, far from **high consciousness** or **good mood** or **well-being**.

Integrative Healing by Marijuana

Healing by Marijuana Therapy is holistic integration of all levels of human experience and all processes of the living organism. It begins with release of the inhibited breath (automatic via interface of cannabis with the body) which then gives rise to rebalancing of the organism as mediated through the ultra-sophistication and great compatibility with exogenous cannabinoids of The Cannabinoid System (not fully understood and only briefly elucidated in this presentation). It is paramount to remember that if the cells are suffocated, the brain is impeded. **There is more not less activity as the organism compensates for the lack** and therefore **fewer spaces and less intervals of molecular and energetic quiet** which feeds into the circle of diminished functioning of the balancing directive of The Cannabinoid System. The envelope of the *mind field* is likewise diminished since it is also affected by insufficiency of the breath. This is a toxic cycle of disease, oftentimes presenting as cancer. The vibrational density of the mental realm as the originating cause of disease furthers its own distortion by inhibited and non-regular *pattern of the breath* borne from the energetic dissonance in the mind field.

The cycle is unremitting without intervention. Once the disease presents, diminished breathing causes yet further distortion. From the mind (*energy field*) surrounding the organism, through the pattern of the breath and then to the body is *the route of manifestation* of disorder. Remediation is most easily accomplished at the level of the breath. The studying of the *volitional* aspect of breathing as opposed to its *automatic* pilot is the key importance of the breath in self-development.

> *Once we know how to contact the Energy of Breath, breathing becomes an infinite source of vitalizing energies*. Kum Nye

Marijuana Therapy has a tradition of thousands of years. It raises the organism to *an altered state* from partial, long-enduring, familiar suffocation to fuller, immediate and unfamiliar oxygenation. The subject is drawn quite predictably and naturally to that which energizes and relaxes simultaneously and which imparts a **good mood** accompanied by a more inclusive, tolerant and profound understanding and which also has noticeable health benefits. Through a boost from plant cannabinoids, The Cannabinoid System becomes re-equipped to carry out its multitudinous functions seen in the microscopic proof of thousands of studies conducted by stringent science. The full potential of human experience is a function of *natural breath* (the birthright of the race) which then sets the agenda for attaining to the heights of health and oftentimes to recognition of the holy. With relaxation of the body and non-worry of the mind, the possibilities for healing are raised to a higher potential.

> *When The Cannabinoid System wears out from over use or improper use, it can be relieved, re-sparked, restarted, and restored by the Primal Cannabinoids of the Ancient Cannabis Sativa.*

The Marijuana Benefit:

As soon as the oil-based Marijuana molecules make contact with the body, there is instant, enthusiastic, electro-magnetic recognition that is experienced with a déjà vu subjectivity not easily put into words. It is a feeling of being uplifted back to the way it seems it once was and should be. In fact, this is the intuitive body/mind remembrance of full breath before the wounds of the world inhibited the constant natural way of breathing. With the infusion of Marijuana into the system, the countless relay stations are re-equipped to carry out the directive from above: Health by Balance mediated by the Hypothalamus region of the brain, which is bathed in cannabinoid receptors. No need to question the effect of Marijuana. It is evidenced in a return to natural balance. Cannabinoids dock to the receptors, thereby activating appropriate processes. They work like passwords. At any moment, hundreds perhaps hundreds of thousands of dockings are taking place. Some result in turning specific computer-stations on; others will be interpreted as holding patterns, and still others produce a shut down or slow down in reactions.

> *The system modulates the excitability and responsiveness of neurons ... by influencing intra-neuronal events, such as the formation of energy providing compounds ... transport of calcium and potassium across the nerve membranes. It undoubtedly interacts with neurotransmitter and neuro-modulator systems. (British Medical Association)*

Lifestyle alone can be held responsible for specifics of imbalance. Tradition wisdom has always taught that irresponsible and/or excessive behaviors destabilize and ultimately damage body/mind.

Modern science has recognized the worn down or burnt out Cannabinoid System that can be and often are re-awakened and restored by the molecules of marijuana. *While the function of the Cannabinoid System is to maintain homeostasis, too often it is overwhelmed*** by the modern habit of continuous stimulation which as citizens of the world, we must all accommodate to whether via healthy coping mechanisms or by the dysfunction of disease. Whether receptors become worn down or the body cannot keep up with the demand for equalizing cannabinoids, the effect of Marijuana on the stressed organism is an immediate re-balancing.

**because of rapid rate of changes ... over the past 150 years, low doses of cannabis should now be regarded as an essential nutrient in order to decrease the toxic level of inflammation that is behind age related illnesses by increasing the homeostatic level of human anti-inflammatory cannabinoid activity. (Melamede)

The Marijuana Remedy:
By the enhancement in the *pattern of the breath* through Marijuana Therapy, fueling of the Cannabinoid System is restored to optimum efficiency from which cellular benefits accrue. Over the course of an **average lifespan, a person takes about 700 million breaths**. Such a practiced habit has far-reaching effects. The *pattern of the breath* takes into account the depth, the silence, the rhythm and the smoothness of inhalation and exhalation and is as subtly unique to each person as a snowflake.

That the unhealthy breather can be retrained is barely incorporated into modern therapy whereas it is essential in Eastern Medicine. Marijuana is **always** healthful if there is even slight diminishment/distress in *the Breath*. In modern society, with the stresses inherent in daily living, no one is exempted from degradation of the breathing process – unless they are super-conscious or completely insulated from the world.

Simply Stated:
Everyone needs to minister to their own worn down Cannabinoid Network (in some way) for the explicit purpose of optimum health!

The net effect of all of the continuous "bindings" within the network of the cannabinoids (more are always being uncovered) to receptors, and including the effects that implicate a non-receptor based effect, is a *chemical event of the most imperceptible, yet far-reaching kind.* Cannabinoids affect all and every system of the organism. Receptors are abundant in the Hypothalamus where autonomic processes are directly connected to/ and impacted by the ubiquitous system whose function is modulation of excitation or balance.

Now we understand from a physiological perspective, why Marijuana Therapy is indicated for daily coping in today's world of extremes. *Cannabinoid Receptors* actually attach to plant cannabinoids with 2 to 3 times more of the affinity to which they attach to the body's own cannabinoids. This is cause for the immediacy of the effects of marijuana and also suggests a connection that is very familiar, comfortable and recognized by body cells as of superior energy. With the addition of Marijuana molecules, there may be more enervation of the Cannabinoid Receptor Network which strangely enough does not suggest more cell activity but may actually translate as a quieting or **toning down** of (re) activity in the service of balance. There may even be an antagonistic effect of the plant cannabinoids to the direction or intensity of the body messages.

The Net Effect of Marijuana
Steadies the Organism.
The Direction Toward Balance
Counteracts the Distortion.

The Balance of Marijuana:
Too much excitation is calmed, excess lethargy is
energized. This personalized *set and setting* effect, is
foolishly considered a detriment of Marijuana Therapy
because it is not a static reaction but instead actually
responds to the real time imbalance of the person.
Marijuana is a Holistic Remedy par excellence which
very naturally resets the organism to its homeostatic
healthful preference. The Western Medical Model is
predicated upon non–individualized, across-the-board
drugging that treats everyone with the same medicine,
regardless of the direction of the distortion. Pain that
arises from tight muscles is different in cause and cure
from neuropathic pain. However, in conventional
medications, numbing the mental or physical discomfort
is the prescription.

To be precise:

With administration of Marijuana:
The body and its surrounding energetic field are
restored to efficacious functioning through
reactivation of the dysfunctional Cannabinoid
Network which then automatically re-balances
the whole person, including the immeasurable
interconnections needed for health (or ease),
thereby allowing the organism to cure itself.

In a Few Words

Quality of the 700 million breaths that serve an average life-span is fundamental to the state of individual health.

Distortion in the *Pattern of the Breath* has immediate as well as long term negative effects.

Marijuana Therapy Restores the Natural Breath.

Marijuana Therapy is the TIMELESS Answer for the Diseases of the Human Race.

Cannabis played a vital role in human evolution thousands of years ago, providing sustenance and solace to the scattered survivors of the great glaciers. It may yet prove to be an equally important asset in our next great evolutionary hurdle as the human race faces the challenge of survival. (Dale Gowin)

Of Interest

In addition, we know that endocannabinoids are not produced when neurons fire just once but only when they fire five or even 10 times in a row.

Scientific facts have proven a bio-physiological primal synchronicity that is reflected in the mental field as well between the microscopic molecules of the ancient co-evolved Marijuana plant and the multi-functional recently discovered Cannabinoid System.

Since these major groundbreaking discoveries, described in a recent interview with Raphael Mechoulam, it appears that dysregulation of the endocannabinoid system is implicated in virtually **all** disease! Its pharmacological modulation holds tremendous promise in treatment of inflammatory, metabolic, and cardiovascular disorders. It is also indicated for pain and cancer. http://www.endocannabinoid.net/Mechoulam.aspx

Conversation with Raphael Mechoulam:
In general, the endocannabinoid system is involved in many different physiological functions, many of which relate to stress-recovery systems and to maintenance of homeostatic balance...other functions: endocannabinoid system- involved in neuro-protection, modulation of nociception, regulation of motor activity and control of certain phases of memory processing. In addition, the endocannabinoid system is involved in modulating the immune/ inflammatory responses. It also influences the cardiovascular and respiratory systems by controlling heart rate, blood pressure, and bronchial functions. Finally, yet importantly, endocannabinoids are known to exert important anti-proliferative actions in tumour cells. (Excerpt from *Addiction*, 2007)

Terpenoids:
Some studies have shown that the odiferous molecular class of compounds of Cannabis Sativa termed the terpenoids may modulate some of the effects of cannabis and may even impact the Endo Cannabinoid System directly. Terpenoids are not unique to cannabis and are abundant in vegetables and fruit.

Chocolate:
A common misconception or *Urban Legend* regarding Marijuana is the presence of cannabinoids in chocolate. That infamous research was never duplicated and is now considered incorrect. But there is an indirect relationship between chocolate and cannabinoids that may clear up the confusion. There are fatty acid derivatives in chocolate as well as in many other plants (including Cannabis Sativa) that inhibit the FAAH (enzyme). FAAH eats Anandamide. Therefore, it is true that if the FAAH Enzyme is inhibited, that process leads to increase/elevation of the body cannabinoid. That's right! Chocolate and the compounds of marijuana both serve the same result allowing for an uptick in cannabinoids throughout the organism. Aspirin has the same effect.

###

At every Progression of The Cancer Biopathy
Opposing Molecular Net Action of Exogenous
Cannabinoids Halts that Progression!

Foreword

When examining modern practices for healthy living, impressive statistics, along with new techniques for viewing old knowledge, promise enduring pleasure and long life. Each scheme has logic, practical methods and convincing sales pitch. Goals are centered exclusively on personal enjoyment without ever suggesting a higher, more global, inclusive perspective. How to enhance whatever experience can be imagined for as long as possible with the least time, cost or effort is the insidious underpinning of the social value, even in the health field. Excess is responsible for infinite diseases of body, mind and spirit yet unending desire is constantly endorsed by the culture which, unfortunately is collectively, subjectively experienced as discontent and always signed by less than full breathing. While Section III is a very brief compilation of the science verifying that *marijuana cures cancer*, commentary is interspersed throughout the evidence from the holistic perspective to make clear that efficient cellular respiration is necessary to *cure* cancer. Even the National Cancer Institute has finally acknowledged the facts:

"The Summary of Marijuana's Medicinal Benefits" was quietly added to the NCI Treatment Plan stating that Oncologists may recommend the intact plant for pain, appetite-stimulation, relaxation and to reduce the size of the tumor: "potential benefits: antiemetic, appetite stimulant, pain relief and improved sleep ... The Health Care Provider may recommend medicinal Cannabis not only for symptom management but also for its possible "ANTI-TUMOUR EFFECT." (3/11)

Introduction

Marijuana is the Fast Path toward Fuller Energy. Marijuana Enhances the Pattern of the Breath Immediately.

The Cancer Biopathy is an outgrowth of a systemic imbalance that proceeds from the *potential toward the tendency and finally to the concrete manifestation of the disease.* It is not an unexpected invasion from outside but just a reaction of the entire personality to what is both within and without. The *potential* refers to the vibration that is invisible but exists nevertheless. It is the living energy of the entity, verified with modern methods, but which is disregarded as irrelevant to the organism's state of health. In fact, when there is a deficit in the energetic envelope that enlivens the person (which can be likened to an insufficiently fueled engine), of course, there is the *tendency* toward transmitting the insufficiency to the mental field and the body, in that order. It is the breath that evidences the primary energetic distortion and it is the habit of the breath that insures the continuance of insufficient energizing. Likewise it is at the level of the breath that there can be the most fundamental alteration toward health.

The mental field accommodates to the energetic habit of breathing which shapes the personality profile of the organism. (The reverse is equally true, i.e., the habit of the breath is the representation of the mental field.) So when it is said that cancer is born in the mind, it is referencing the *tendency toward* the Cancer Biopathy, defined by the way a person breathes, thinks, eats and generally copes. It is not so much a prediction, but more a probability considering the many other contributory variables. Nonetheless, for the cancer-prone individual, life challenges often seem overwhelming. Rather than deep breathing and a casual relaxed attitude, low level anxiety (suffocation) persists even in safe settings.

56

Not fully exhaling *emanates from and creates* an undercurrent of tension in the mind and in the muscles. By dissolving the tension that is a subjective background to all that is played out on the life stage, **marijuana reverses the tendency toward the Cancer Biopathy.** Unfortunately, the modern medical profession has no understanding of preventive measures for health and less inclination to intervene before a disturbance has evolved from the probable to the actual. It does not deal in abstracts. The numbers tell the story. If tests from the *up-to-the-minute diagnostic equipment* are within *"acceptable-range,"* regardless of life style, warning signs or reported discomforts, the doctor assigns the status of a *clean bill of health.* The patient is validated to continue breathing, eating, drinking, thinking as usual probably with the addition of some not-**so**-lethal depressant prescribed for the original complaint. On the other hand, when imbalance is red-flagged, the doctor intervenes aggressively, perhaps with drugs to mask the symptoms and further on down the line with even more dangerous treatment procedures.

Today's mindset has doctors administering immediate relief for every symptom. Incredibly, the cause is unrelated to the treatment. Science does not address the vibrational reality that exists in universal processes. Any energetic forewarning that foretells the concrete presentation of disease is not recognized. Medicine is based on technology that measures gross instability. Objective science prides itself on not looking beyond what can be measured and therefore cannot know that a vibrational deficiency pre-dates what is finally a progressed degradation to the physical plane. With that basic unwavering orientation and despite the bias against all things that smack of traditional "folk-lore," **medical science has itself proven** the **Benefits of Marijuana** with intricate almost comedic detail.

Although still in denial of the concrete reality of a higher order of being than the material, by its own stringent scientific research it is clear that Marijuana Therapy is a holistic remedy that impacts the three levels of human existence: the material, the mental and the subtle energetic realm expressed in the habit of the breath. Cancer is the *disease classification* assigned to material expression of energetic disturbance. The potential becomes the actual. From the undetected weakness in the energy matrix that defines the cancer personality; without intervention for expanding the limited breath, the process of cancer is completed on the physical plane. At this stage, the physical component of the entity is visibly dysfunctional and/or damaged. The derangement can no longer be ignored. Action is mandated if the possibility of health is to be recaptured. To change the atmosphere and/or whatever unhealthful and entrenched habits of daily living caused the sickness in the first place, interest and wise action are called for, both of which are in short supply in the frantic days that follow the fateful diagnosis of cancer. Enter the cellular restorative benefits of the cannabinoids of Marijuana.

Balancing of Marijuana Therapy

The Theoretical:
From the viewpoint of holistic healing, the therapeutic objective in all disease is to re-ignite the complex, interrelationship of all the energetic and bio/chemical connections so that the body, mind and invisible vibrational field are in sync which will automatically disengage any symptom borne of disharmony. At the *biological level*, optimum health expresses high level cooperation and unencumbered communication in the cells. It is now clear that when The Cannabinoid System is operating at peak performance, it maintains order in all body processes by allowing no undue **chronic excitation or inflammation**.

But if this ubiquitous multi-tasking signaling system becomes exhausted, worn out, ineffective or in any way unreliable, the entity develops problems in all areas. The mechanics behind derailing the Cannabinoid System from its usual aplomb have not been studied at all. In the science of the Holistic Philosophy, it is apparent that chronic suffocation is the original deprivation that injures the basic mechanism of balance. Envisioning the moment-to-moment super activity that defines the society from the very first natural inspiration until the last limited exhalation conjures up a harried lifetime struggle. Although, in modern industrialized nations, daily existence is not usually threatened, the human mind creates its own dangers mirrored in the physical chemicals that stress our bodies.

Constant activity, self-concern, competitive attitudes, and including toxic diets and unwholesome activities are not upheld by the healthy breath. There is almost not enough time to breathe and certainly not enough relaxation of the entity. Not being able to accommodate to full oxygenation, translates as weakness or deficiency in the mechanism of balance. In addition, the endogenous Cannabinoids are made on demand to accommodate to whatever need presents. If there is excess need (owing to lifestyle) along with insufficient oxygenation, dysregulation of the entire network predictably ensues. *(Factors not covered in this presentation, but relevant when searching out environmental causes for cancer: the increasingly poisoned and de-oxygenated atmosphere adds more problems to the faulty habit of breathing; and unhealthy food, having to do with poor habit as well as the collective degradation of the food supply.)*

Once The Cannabinoid System loses its ability to modulate, regulate and balance the organism, non-cooperation persists in groupings of recalcitrant cells that no longer resonate with the rhythm of the whole. To restore homeostasis, a gentle, natural and non-injurious coaxing is required.

The Practical:
The results of scientific tests are full of fine detail that point to an incredible multitude of processes that are either restored or implemented with compounds of Marijuana; and which are derivative to a general re-oxygenation of the entity. Almost every other day, a new study is published that proves the palliative, preventive, and curative aspects of Marijuana. Thousands of studies from around the globe have demonstrated very many and varied anti-cancerous effects from compounds of Cannabis Sativa, such as that Lung Cancer is prevented within statistically significant limits in the general population; Breast and Prostate Cancer, some Blood Cancer and Brain Cancer, etc., are all stopped at some stage in the Cancer Biopathy by Marijuana Therapy (in some form or another). The specific findings (in the following pages) prove that complex cellular interactions that become dysfunctional during cancer are rejuvenated by plant cannabinoids.

The General:
As noted: The most noticeable (and measurable) result from the intake of marijuana is increased volume per breath. That is, marijuana expands and enhances the breathing process. Out from this simple but life-affirming effect, efficiency in body processing is greatly improved, expressed as well in increased mental clarity.

Some interesting data was available nearly half a century ago that demonstrated the extent of the breath facilitation that takes place with administration of marijuana, but unfortunately, any further studies have not been forthcoming and those old results were long ago shelved and are no longer accessible. However, in the 70s, before the ban on studying any benefits of marijuana, research with healthy subjects demonstrated a 40% decrease in resistance in the large airway with the administration of smoked marijuana. Simultaneously, an increase of nearly 50% in airway conductance was observed. Personally, I have detailed notes from these studies but alas, the underground source is lost to time.

In other words, those studies (that have not been authenticated by modern science – yet!) demonstrate that chronic, habitual muscle holding, along with the habitual lack of deep breathing which limits the life experience was diminished by nearly 50% with marijuana. Simultaneously, actual air conducted was increased by 50%. No such studies were conducted on patients with chronic disease, but the logical expectation is that aeration would be at least as much improved. There is no doubt that these tests will be replicated within current parameters and that the findings will be similarly stunning. It is just a matter of time before the entire medical community is inundated with the vast array of the benefits of Marijuana.

As a Healing Agent specific to the Chaos of Cancer Marijuana Compounds Fulfill the Prime Directive:
CAUSE NO HARM
While Re-Sparking the Natural Order

Choosing Marijuana is *The Healthy Choice*:
Stress is a major hurdle for the collective global population in the midst of the insecurity of modern life. Ways of coping include all sorts of activities, many of which are detrimental to the organism in the long run. Those who opt to gain freedom of breath, such as with spiritual practice, breathing exercises, and/or the naturally beneficial Cannabis Sativa are instinctively opting for health. To exhale stagnant air and to inhale deeply, rather than becoming angry and constricted in the face of frustration marks the impulse toward well-being. Millions of people in all walks of life, from all nations, in all age brackets find that marijuana melts their muscular tension, easily, safely and almost immediately while making room for a breath of fresh air that literally wafts throughout the organism and allows for exhaling the accumulated energetic necrosis along with fear and frustration. That is *The Marijuana Effect of Expanding the Mind and Raising the Consciousness.*

Marijuana deepens the breath, smoothes calms and quiets it. Muscles throughout the entire body, including the oppositional muscles that contain the chest relax dramatically allowing for the lungs to swell in dimension and capacity. More than any other healing effect from Marijuana, expansion of the capillaries in the lungs is by far the most profound. In addition, as a direct consequence of administering Marijuana, many specific chemical interchanges are seen that demonstrate anti-cancerous activity. From the thousands of studies over the last few decades, the major conclusions are:
1) Cannabinoids are Selective Anti-Tumor Compounds;
2) Cannabinoids Kill Tumors;
3) Cannabinoids Do Not Damage Healthy Cells.

It should be borne in mind that the integrative and inherent cellular anti-cancer actions of the exogenous cannabinoids have been tested as single isolated molecules, in artificial circumstances. The boundless synergy of action that is continuously occurring in the entire organism and among the limitless combinations of body and plant cannabinoids is generally not realized. Certainly the profound *holistic* benefits of marijuana are under-appreciated and for the most part, not understood. Recently, Pacific Medical Center researchers stated:

1) Cannabinoids *possess Synergistic Anti-Cancer Properties;*
2) Combined *Plant Constituents are Superior to Isolated Compounds;*
3) Recommendation for Cancer Therapy: *At least add Cannabidiol, with one other cannabinoid.*

Adding back one more cannabinoid to a genus with over 500 is definitely a tiny, tiny step in the logic of healing. Not to incorporate all 499 ingredients sadly points to a commercial motive. But reality is dawning. Capitulation to the truth by the NCI may really signal a change toward liberation as the truth becomes more public.

Prevention is Best:
The review that follows deals with already advanced stages of cancer, understood as having become obvious enough for a diagnosis within the parameters of Western Medicine. The fact remains, however, that the visible manifestation is but the end result of reaching the tipping point of cell-suffocation. Better not to arrive at this stage where the potential toward the specific illness is realized on the physical plane.

**Marijuana Therapy Prevents Diseases of Imbalance.
Cancer is the Ultimate Imbalance**

It is absolutely true and scientifically documented:
At every stage in the progression of the Cancer Biopathy there is a dysfunctional molecular reaction that once restored by the Exogenous cannabinoids halts the progression of cancer at that stage. **This is not a mystery. It is a medical miracle**. It is also remarkably misunderstood. There is no doubt that the intact plant is preventive for stress-caused illnesses. Prevention is Best! It is surely better to alter the habit that results in a life-endangering disease before (and not after) the organism has succumbed to the illness.

Extracted and/or Synthetic Cannabinoids:
Results with Cannabis are mostly based on aggressive, technology. Extracted compounds from the Cannabis Plant or synthetic facsimiles of just a few cannabinoids have been administered by injection. Both in vivo and in vitro results have been noteworthy and newsworthy! The extracted, single molecules of Marijuana have in fact resulted in cancer regression. Unfortunately, hardly any studies have been conducted where the natural, intact plant was compared to the unnatural single molecule administration of a particular cannabinoid (or two). However, one very recent study stands out as an amazing validation for the benefits of inhaled Marijuana as they pertain to The Cancer Biopathy as it presents in Brain Cancer.

(Mansoor Foroughi PhD is the leading author of hopefully the first of many scientific papers (2011) reporting that **smoked Marijuana** was responsible for the spontaneous regression of gliomas (*Brain Cancer*). The conclusion: while there may well be need for aggressive treatment with concentrated extracted and injected cannabinoids in the face of imminent threat to life, there are times that call for the natural plant. (Why such easily designed comparisons have not been conducted becomes a point of interest and suspicion.)

The studies show how different cannabinoids work as anti-cancer agents on deranged cells utilizing just one or two isolated marijuana compounds or synthetic versions of cannabinoids. Results have demonstrated benefits at every stage of the material progression of cancer.

The Question Remains: *Why is there such a dearth of public information concerning whether or not and in what possible way copious amounts of Marijuana might prevent or cure cancer? (Part IV offers some answers.)*

Cellular Benefits of Marijuana Therapy:

It is clear that enhanced breathing begins a revitalizing process to the constricted organism. It should be clear that sickness and poor breathing go hand-in-hand. The healing that follows re-oxygenation in various observed instances of utilizing Marijuana is also clear. It has been recorded in numerous, seemingly custom-tailored bio-chemical studies. Actions of plant cannabinoids proceed to impede or completely disrupt cancer progression and development. These definitely favorable actions are documented by scientists over and over all around the world and reported in-depth over the last decade in scientific journals and also in cyber-space, but hardly ever to the mainstream audience.

This unquestionable scientifically gathered evidence over the last decade is synopsized in the following pages geared specifically to the lay reader with brief commentary to make stunningly clear how marijuana prevents and cures, not just the expression of The Cancer Biopathy but also the predisposition toward the dread disease.

#1 Non-Proliferation - Tumor Cells Disabled:
(Growth Inhibited, Tumor is Inhibited)

In a definitive study with Marijuana and breast cancer, the extremely aggressive cancer cells that usually over-grow the host organ and spread through the system stopped being replicated when just one of the 60 or so marijuana cannabinoids was administered. That is, in breast cancer cells, the Marijuana compound, CBD, stopped the expression of a particularly dangerous gene before it was transcribed or before its reproduction/ replication. Once cancer tissue becomes prevalent, the prime directive of the organism and the healer is to stop it. Whereas chemo kills the cancer cells, it does so at the expense of healthy tissue. But Marijuana compounds have been demonstrated to halt the cancer quite definitely and without compromising healthy cells. In addition, simultaneously and as a contributor to disrupting the progression of cancer, Marijuana allows for the full and natural breathing that encourages the **body** to regain equilibrium and health.

CBD ...first non-toxic Exogenous agent (to) decrease Id-1 expression in metastatic breast cancer ...leading to down-regulation of tumor-aggressiveness. (McAllister)

The above quote by a noted researcher demonstrates the propaganda that is still so difficult to overcome. THC (NOT CBD) was the first cannabinoid to decrease metastasis in breast cancer. Shamefully, the truth about the magic molecule was hidden from the media, the public and the patients for over a quarter of a century and acknowledged only after the conclusive study was found in the archives of a library. The suggestion that THC (or any Plant Cannabinoid) IS TOXIC is A 100% contradiction of 5000 years of experience and thousands of modern scientific studies.

Time-tested herbals are devalued in the industrial era even though it is less than a century since legal, one-directional designer Drugs (often with killing side effects) replaced naturally balancing, safe Botanicals. As for the Cannabis Plant, science has proven that leaves, stalk, root and flowers and all compounds that comprise its resins are imbued with natural balancing compounds for the human organism, none of which are dangerous or in the least bit harmful. To suggest otherwise is to be ignorant or disingenuous. Further to imply that harm issues from the high feeling, or *"a sense of well-being"* is to disregard and disrespect the major conclusion of the definitive study by The Institute of Medicine. It stated categorically, that the *"high itself"* or *"the good mood consciousness might be curative"* and that Plant cannabinoids had the effects of *moderation, modulation and regulation!!!!*

This prestigious agency weighed its words carefully and deserves great credit, especially to the authors of the study who were so forthcoming with the truth despite opposing political agendas. Unfortunately, mainstream News Media chose not to publicize the momentous findings. It is a fact that as we go forward into the second decade of the 21rst century, the *high feeling* is still deemed a negative by the establishment. Sadly, untruthful and misleading information is still given the stamp of approval:

> *The psychotropic effects of Δ9-THC and additional cannabinoid agonists, mediated through CB1 Receptor, LIMIT their clinical utility. CBD does not have appreciable affinity for the CB1 or CB2 Receptors and does not have psychotropic activities.*

Inhibitory action of CBD from Cannabis Sativa on metastatic breast cancer is fully acknowledged! It is preferred to THC by the medical profession because it imparts **no high**. Its bio-chemical interactions within the tumour occur through unknown pathways, accomplished outside the usual network. This unique action suggests even more processes for exogenous cannabinoids that are anti-cancerous.

Regardless of the specifics of their cellular activity, whether within or without usual channels, research shows that cannabinoids (body or plant) with or without the wonderful **side effect of a good mood, inhibit proliferation** of many types of cancers:

> *Breast cancer, prostate-cancer, cervical and colorectal carcinoma, brain cancer (glioma), gastric adeno-carcinoma / skin cancer uterine cancer / thyroid epithelioma lymphoma and pancreatic-adeno-carcinoma.*

That is, whatever type cancer has so far been studied has responded favourably to Marijuana Therapy. No doubt the trend will continue, promising even more varied proofs. The possibility seems closer than ever before when the *high* feeling will be elevated to a superior position on the continuum of healing.

#2 *Apoptosis (Suicide by Marijuana):*

Even though each anti-cancer activity that is measured in the body is seen as a sequential and isolated event, in fact, the array of processes that arise automatically to combat sick cells is multi-tasking and integrative. It is only in discussion that separation exists.

The action called *Apoptosis* is none other than deformed cells dying quite routinely as a function of maintaining the integrity of the whole. They commit suicide rather than contaminating the barrel! More than any other action singled out for study, *Apoptosis* can be said to be in keeping with the homeostatic mandate. Survival of the whole comes at the cost of non-survival of a part. From a psychological perspective, cancer can be described as selfish cells that struck out on their own when the going got tough and the oxygenation became deficient instead of committing the ultimate sacrifice. Non- nourished components are predictably not in sync with the major plan.

In contrast, in the healthy (aerated) organism, *Apoptosis* functions as fundamental to the on-going agenda. The cellular composite shares in cooperative communication so that no part of the organism is neglected or denied. All components are nurtured. Visible manifestation of cellular synchrony is expressed also psychologically. The reverse is true as well where chronic mental distress (however hidden) is manifest physically.

Cancer personality profiles are often described as not loving (the whole of) themselves. Emotions are contained. Anger is dismissed. The breath is deficient. Cells are deprived. Rebellion is Inevitable. When the personality is at odds with itself, the body is a corporeal mirror-image of that state. Rather than incorporation of all attributes of the individual, a selective façade is adopted. "Certain emotions "are stuffed,"

Not acknowledging what is felt can often produce chronically starved *areas of unconsciousness,* evidenced and exacerbated by insufficiency in the habit of the breath with associated mental/physical problems. These features are subtle and not considered relevant in conventional treatments for cancer, even though these features are constant throughout the life experience. Without purposeful and appropriate intervention, the lacking in integration of the personality is always impacting the expression of cancer in the cells owing to the deficit in respiration. This is the description of a vicious toxic circle (VTC) that is self propelling.

With the all-encompassing distress from the fear of the cancer diagnosis; the discomfort and pain caused by medical treatments; as well as the depressant drugs to limit pain, breathing actually becomes more restricted and more insufficient. In conventional medicine, cancer treatments too often become the vehicle by which a patient's health spirals downward rather than toward health, which is in absolute opposition to fundamentals of Holistic Science, geared always toward re-instating oxygenation throughout the organism.

Marijuana is a Facilitator of *The Breath*

In cases of spontaneous remission, it is interesting to note, that the psychological orientation itself seems to lighten. Reports from recovered patients refer to a reversal in attitude that frees them to accept who they really are; to be honest in relationships; to take charge of challenges, without resorting to sweeping them under the rug. Liberation of the mind corresponds with a relaxation in the muscles and in the habit of the breath. In those rare cases of unexplained recovery, it is clear that repression has given way to resolution. While no formal studies are imagined to measure expansion in respiration and correlation to spontaneous remissions, in fact, the relationship is a truism.

70

Alteration of the cancer personality toward health defines less repressed breathing. Psychologically, the person is in tune with herself so that experiences can be frontal without shying away from feelings. Physically, the body is in cellular harmony. Deficient cells that do not answer the self-destruct mandate meet the next anti-cancer check-point by responding to Anti-proliferation signals. That is, when the operation of the autonomic processes have become realigned by not being so suffocated, if a sick cell forgets to self-destruct, the next checkpoint will act as quality control and the unhealthy cells will not proliferate.

Examined as different processes, in fact the two anti-cancer actions of *non-proliferation* and *apoptosis* are married in real cell life.

Marijuana Restores Respiration to Efficient Functioning. Natural Healing is Recharged.

Extracted THC Decreases the (*livingness of*) Tumor: Significant increases in programmed cell death have been accomplished in vitro with the administration of just **one** Marijuana compound. Testing conducted on mice who were first infected with cancer cells and then injected with THC clearly demonstrated that the *numbers of tumors decreased significantly while the activity of Apoptosis increased*, resulting in less tumors and less production of tumors. Harkening back to homeostasis was simultaneously evoked. The cells responded to the directive of survival of the whole and no longer to the separatist call of the Cancer Biopathy.

End Result: Mice given THC lived significantly longer.

It is apparent that the process of *Apoptosis is restored with Marijuana compounds* which automatically reactivate the suicide mandate for the individual cell. Indeed, cancerous cells respond very quickly to the plant cannabinoids of Marijuana. Apoptosis began as soon as six hours from the time that THC was first administered to leukemia cells!

Closely involved with the self destruct of unhealthy cells by *Apoptosis*, is yet another process: *Autophagy*. As its name implies, it is self-digestion of deranged cells, (certainly complementary to *Apoptosis*). In fact, *Autophagy* might just be the beginning stage of the self-destruct of Apoptosis.

Regardless, Natural THC encourages both processes!

Anti-cancer activity is dependent upon the modulation of key signaling-pathways that trigger cancer cell death (and it was) recently observed that THC induces glioma cell death through stimulation of *Autophagy*. *Autophagy* is upstream of Apoptosis in THC-induced cancer-cell death and activation of this pathway is necessary for the THC anti-cancer action. (Guzman et al)

> **Programmed Cell Death (*Apoptosis*):
> REBOOTED by *The Marijuana Effect***

#3 Tumours Shrink with Injection of THC

Nearly two decades ago, Madrid Complutense University published results demonstrating that THC was able to shrink aggressive brain tumours (gliomas). In 1998 The Journal FEBS Letters reported that the infamous THC cannabinoid induced *apoptosis* in gliomas (in culture). By the turn of the century, yet more research was conducted by combining extracted THC molecules from the plant with a synthetic cannabinoid. The observed results acknowledged "considerable regression of malignant gliomas (in animals.)" Those findings were confirmed with yet another study. But because THC suffers from the stigma of the *high feeling*, scientists continued to search. They extracted the CBD cannabinoid (it has no High effect) and it demonstrated considerable anti-tumour activity on gliomas (*in vitro* and *in vivo*). These studies could not be conducted in the U.S. since all studies that hypothesize a benefit to Marijuana are banned.

There is a voluminous body of work that has been conducted outside of America that reveals the general, widespread advantages of **healing, calming, curing and palliating the symptoms of cancer,** and other life-endangering diseases **with Marijuana Therapy** but it is mostly hidden from the lay population. Although clinical tests with: *extracted plant cannabinoids*; with *synthetic cannabinoids*; and *with a combination of the two* have all shown *very positive results in shrinking tumours of the brain* **and** there are amazing testimonials of Marijuana shrinking cancerous brain tumours and saving lives of terminally ill patients – no studies are in the planning stages to test natural Marijuana as a remedy. Pharmaceutical companies keep extracting and testing since research with natural Cannabis Sativa is not conducive to profit and therefore not planned.

There is no doubt that *cannabinoids... act as anti-neoplastic agents. Cannabinoids* prevent, inhibit or halt development of a tumor/neoplasm, *particularly on glioma cell lines.* There is no question with any of the findings. Cannabinoids inhibit glioma tumor growth in animals and humor tumor samples *by altering blood vessel morphology.* (Guzman)

Constituents of Marijuana are 1) anti-cancerous; and 2) selective in action. Cannabinoids cause cancerous tissue to lose nourishment, while healthy cells juxtaposed to the cancer are not affected! But chemotherapy cannot discriminate and kills healthy as well as sick tissue. On a positive note, there just may be an inkling of recognizing the benefits of Marijuana: ***"Medical science now supports combination therapy" such as extracted Plant Cannabinoids combined with conventional anti-cancer drugs!"*** As noted: 2011 saw the NCI (arm of a government agency) add a **"summary of marijuana's medicinal benefits"** to its recommended treatments, even encouraging oncologists to recommend (intact) Marijuana for pain, nausea and depression.

This was/is pretty BIG NEWS but it did not make the News. Nevertheless the announcement was public, hidden in small print where it might not be noticed and also posted via internet.

The potential benefits of medicinal Cannabis for people living with cancer include: antiemetic effects, appetite-stimulation, pain relief and improved sleep. In the practice of integrative oncology, the health care provider may recommend medicinal Cannabis not only for symptom management but also for possible direct antitumor effects. (NCI, 2011)

Regardless of its threat to the major pharmaceutical complex, *The **Intelligence of Marijuana*** is too powerful to contain. With just one or possibly two of its over 500 plus compounds, still Marijuana enhances fueling to healthy tissue. Simultaneously, cancerous tissue loses its source of nourishment. There is less vascularization to the tumor following Marijuana administration. (3/11)

> *There is less inflammation in surrounding tissue... safety profile of THC with possible anti-proliferative action on tumors **may** set the stage to evaluate anti-tumor action of cannabinoids.* (http://norml.org/index.cfm?Group_ID=7008).

The facts behind these studies present an astoundingly positive profile for the administration of THC and perhaps another isolated cannabinoid or two: Less inflammation in the tissue next to the tumor; a great safety profile; and the tumor shrinks. What more could we want? But the wonderfully positive results do not guarantee interest or investigation. Instead, evidence that Marijuana destroys cancerous tissue has the scientific community only slightly interested and it has stated that it just *"MAY EVALUATE"* the anti-tumor- action of cannabinoids. Why not immediately for sure?

Spontaneous Regression:
Well it seems that fate has intervened into the politically restricted arena of science by gifting the citizens of the world with a wondrous example of healing by *inhaled Marijuana for Brain Cancer*. This documentation was not a controlled study, but was instead the ongoing monitoring of two teenage women with brain tumors. Consequential shrinking of the tumors was not within usual scientific parameters, leading researchers to delve further into the details. M. Foroughi, PhD. published the unprecedented results of two female cancer patients with an unusual acknowledgement: ***Marijuana Inhalation May Keep Brain Cancer in Remission!*** (March 2011)

Two girls (11 and 14) underwent surgery for gliomas (brain cancer). A six year follow-up showed both tumors shrank significantly without explanation/expectation. Investigation resulted in admission by both girls of the *Marijuana Lifestyle* of many teens:

Patient stated: she began smoking cannabis at 14 when first diagnosed, and continued daily from 16 to 19 years of age. As they scanned her brain over the course of time, the tumor mass became smaller with each checkup (almost gone after six years). The story was the same for both girls and the only explanation was the *Variable of inhaling Cannabis*. In another era, this study might easily be misplaced purposely. Thankfully, that cannot happen today. Especially with the speed and breadth of modern communication, the public cannot be kept in the dark. This is a very big crack in the iceberg and is almost an admission that *Marijuana cures cancer*.

Foroughi and his team, in an exceptional and politically incorrect display of logic have even suggested that there *may be plant synergy* among all the compounds of Cannabis Sativa and recommend studying the whole plant: "Since any beneficial effect may not be caused by one compound, molecule or cannabinoid alone."

#4 _Metastasis:_
(Stopped in its tracks with Marijuana Therapy)

After the initial shock, the first question a patient asks when given the dread diagnosis is "Can you catch it in time? The meaning is simple: has it/ can it/ and/or will it spread? The research is definite: _Anandamide when_ administered (injected) alone or in combination with Plant cannabinoids has shown anti-cancer spreading effects. In fact, when Endogenous cannabinoids are compared to EXogenous cannabinoids for tumor suppression/anti-invasiveness, molecules from the Plant were quite a bit more effective. Anandamide scored only between 38 and 84% effectiveness in its suppression ability, while natural THC ranged from 69 to 104%. (The study used cervical cancer (HeLa) cells and lung carcinoma cells (A549).

> _Plant Cannabinoids_ **may** ... _offer therapeutic treatment of highly invasive cancers._ (J Nat. Cancer Inst., 2008) _As we have seen ... over-expression of the Id-1 gene caused the tumor to grow. (It has been proven that) Marijuana suppresses Id-1 which suppresses nourishment, growth and spreading of cancer cells._ (ibid)

Studies on all phases of the anti-cancer action of marijuana have been conducted in many other countries. A German study made the discovery that CBD seems to have another pathway: **an unknown mechanism** _that helps its anti-cancer action especially in metastasis: underlying the Anti-Invasive Action of Cannabidiol on Human Lung Cancer and an_ **anti-invasive action** _of cannabidiol on human lung cancer cells."_ (Ramer R, et al. 2010 _Jul 29._) In fact, with the administration of just one or two of Plant cannabinoids, the tumor stops growing and shrinks! Cancerous cells die automatically.

Metastasis Cannot Proceed.

#5 Anti-Inflammatory:
(Calming By Marijuana)

Does it all really start here? Is Inflammation the First Dysfunction of the Deprived Cell?

When it comes to the anti-inflammatory properties of Marijuana, everyone be assured that they exist; are extremely effective; very unique and very valuable. This is an ABSOLUTE CERTAINTY because in 2003, the **United States Government** applied and was granted a **Patent on the Anti-Inflammatory Properties of the Cannabis Sativa Plant!** Patent **#6,630,507** was issued and also covered neuro-protective features of the plant. This information was NOT publicized as the prohibition mentality was/is still in place. In addition, the patent refers to the effectiveness of inhaled Marijuana:

> The Department of Health and Human Services was awarded a patent on the "medical benefits of cannabinoids," derived from the natural plant. (based on studies of the National Institute of Health which also have not been publicized.)

On Oct 7, 2003, U.S. Patent No. 6, 630,507 was issued: *Cannabinoids as Antioxidants and Neuroprotectants.* A. Hampson, J. Axelrod and M. Grimaldi are listed as the Inventors of the properties of the plant! The patent covers cannabinoids for: *Oxidation-associated Disease* and *Neuro-Degenerative Disease.* The literature refers quite brazenly to the excellent absorption of compounds via Inhalation. (*Inhaled Route*)

> *Cannabinoids are neuro-protectants and anti-inflammatory* and as such are useful in the prevention and treatment and as such are useful in the prevention and treatment of a wide variety of diseases including stroke, trauma, auto-immune disorders, Parkinson's, Alzheimer's and HIV. (Science Daily, Apr. 17, 2007)

78

Inflammation is actually a reasonable coping mechanism for starving cells. More blood and stimulation to a trauma site makes sense. But with chronic insufficiency, inflammation itself becomes the illness causing damage over the long term. When at first, you don't succeed, try, try again and again. Deprived cells as well as depressed personalities tend to follow this circle of desperate behavior which contributes to inflammation, very conducive to developing cancer. When the natural feedback of the organism becomes disoriented, The Cannabinoid System is stressed. Cellular instructions to cease a particular cascade of processes (or not) are lost, ignored, or never sent because the usual equalizing operations of the Cannabinoid Network are not working. *Endo-Cannabinoid Deficiency Syndrome* (ECDS) is the new term to describe the imbalance which consequently destabilizes the organism. According to Raphael Mechoulam:

> *Dysregulation of the endo-cannabinoid system may be implicated in virtually **all diseases.** Its pharmacological modulation holds tremendous promise (for) inflammatory, metabolic, and cardiovascular disorders, also pain and cancer.*

Cannabinoids have the Natural Ability to Modulate in Step-Wise Fashion the Over-Excited Cellular Chaos That Occurs in the Cancer Cycle.

Administration of cannabinoids from Marijuana evokes direct and remarkably rapid restoration to functionality. The healing effect is evident. If there is hyper-stimulation, it is simply **toned down**. The reverse is equally true. The Compounds of Cannabis Sativa (and some synthetic *cannabimemetics*) stop tumor growth by accessing, impacting and re-righting the dysfunctional and/or defunct multi-action biochemical pathways within and around cancerous cells.

#6 Lung Cancer Findings:
Science has Proven the Opposite of the Propaganda!

The Amazing Fact:
Marijuana Cuts Lung Cancer Tumour Growth in Half reported in Science Daily **three+ years ago** but was hardly a news flash in the repressed media. Only those interested in the benefits of Marijuana were in the e-loop of this amazing knowledge.

"The active ingredient in marijuana cuts tumour growth in common lung cancer in half and significantly reduces the ability of the cancer to spread. THC inhibited growth and spread...researchers do not know why THC inhibits tumour growth but they speculate that (it) could be activating molecules that arrest the cell cycle and ... THC may interfere with angiogenesis and vascularization, which promotes cancer growth." (Harvard, Science Daily, 2007)

Believe it or not, this was not big news in the "**in** circle" because it was really old news. Back in 1975 the *anti-cancer effects of cannabis in Lewis Lung Tumours* were proven (Munson). The study was government funded. The hypothesis was that Marijuana damaged the Immune System. But the opposite was inconveniently proven. Marijuana was shrinking the cancerous tumours. It actually stopped the body from producing *cancerous cells*. The *anti-proliferative* action of Marijuana on cancer cells was discovered. What happened next is not believable! First of all the study was shelved by the government. It was not rediscovered until some astute activists searched out the archives 30 or so years later. From that momentous discovery: ***Marijuana Cured Breast Cancer*** until now, all studies on any benefits of Marijuana were banned by the U.S. government. What else can hiding the truth from endangered patients be called except criminal?

To Clarify this Criminal Action:
Once the incredibly promising anti-cancer benefits of Marijuana were scientifically confirmed, all research aimed at discovering any health benefits from Cannabis Sativa were outlawed by the U.S. government! Only tests by Pharmaceutical Companies were allowed and those agencies never tested the benefits of the intact Marijuana plant. Research consists of dissecting and copying an ingredient or two of the complex Cannabis Sativa Plant for commercial drug preparation. (No studies on the intact plant are even planned.) The Mega Industry continues to search for the silver bullet, characteristically out of sync with the merciful flower's gentle tendency toward healing while the effective ancient remedy is obscured by the propaganda of profit.

Fortunately, in many other countries, thousands of serious studies proving the benefits of Marijuana are slowly overtaking the misinformation. In 1998, the body cannabinoid (*Anandamide*) was tested on breast cancer. It exhibited definite anti-proliferative effects. Over the past few decades, continuing research has resulted in a varied wealth of knowledge concerning **ex**ogenous and **en**dogenous cannabinoid effects. Conclusions have all been positive and the literature abounds with research demonstrating unparalleled versatility of cannabinoids which often utilize unknown biological pathways in their anti-cancer arsenal of tricks.

One telling study was reported in Science Daily in 2007. Mice were implanted with human lung cancer cells and then injected with THC. The stunning results are still circulating on the internet, but no change has occurred in U.S. Policy and the story hardly made mainstream news.

> Science Daily (April 17, 2007): *The active ingredient in marijuana cuts tumour growth in common lung cancer in half and significantly reduces the ability of the cancer to spread.*

The conclusions of the researchers were predictable. Rather than looking into the intact natural and ancient remedy, the mode of exploitation maintains: *The beauty of this study is that we are showing that a **substance of abuse**, if used prudently, may offer a new road to therapy against lung cancer*, Division of Experimental Medicine, (A. Preet, Ph.D., noted Cannabinoid scientist)

Marijuana Diminished Tumor Size: (by 50%)
In the Control Group, cancers continued to develop. But Not in the Marijuana Group:

> *(There was) evidence of a sixty percent (60%) reduction in cancer lesions of the lungs,* and also there was *a statistically significant reduction in (protein) markers pointing to cancer.* Scientists speculate: *THC may interfere with angiogenesis and tumor vascularization.*

Even with such spectacular data, hardly anyone in the for-Profit Health Professions admits being impressed.

> *much work is needed to clarify pathway by which THC functions... data support the further testing of cannabidiol and cannabidiol-rich extracts for the potential treatment of cancer.* (ibid)

> *In conclusion, our data indicate that cannabidiol and possibly Cannabis extracts enriched in this natural cannabinoid represent a **promising non-psychoactive and anti-neoplastic strategy**. In particular, for a **highly malignant human breast carcinoma cell line, we have shown here that cannabidiol and a cannabidiol-rich extract counteract cell growth both in vivo and in vitro as well as tumor metastasis in vivo.***" (ibid.)

Actually, the Lung Cancer Study conducted by Tashkin and funded by the U.S. Government itself tops all the conclusions thus far. The hypothesis was simply that Marijuana caused Lung Cancer. Instead, the results demonstrated without doubt both healing and preventive benefits from Marijuana. Dr. Donald Tashkin conducted a 30 year study of over 1000 subjects. He found that in comparison to heavy tobacco smokers who had a 20% higher incidence of Pulmonary Diseases, even *heavy marijuana smokers* (of 30+ years) had no abnormality in lung function whatsoever! Heavy Marijuana smokers actually showed a higher degree of health than the control group who did not smoke!! His conclusions:

> There is **no link** between marijuana smoke and lung cancer, including long-term and abusive smoking. Instead, there is a positive effect for marijuana users. THC has Anti-proliferative, Anti-carcinogenic and Apoptosis Effects.

http://www.youtube.com/watch?v=_6pBw0bgmgA, and http://www.sciencedaily.com/releases/2006/05/060526083353.htm

This protection is an organic response. It does not take place in a test tube which is where so many prior studies were held which suggested that Marijuana somehow was carcinogenic. In fact, the inorganic material of the test-tube cannot interface with the smoke of Marijuana via the inherent protective molecular action between plant cannabinoids and The Cannabinoid System of a live subject. In other words, although there is carcinogenic particulate matter in Marijuana smoke, the Anti-Cancer effects of marijuana neutralize any potential damage.

Of course, the hypothesis of the Tashkin study was that marijuana and cigarettes were both cancer-causing. But the truth prevailed. What was demonstrated was the absolute fact and great dismaying surprise that even heavy Marijuana smokers enjoyed reduced incidence of Lung Cancer when compared to the general population.

And while nicotine causes lung cancer, without a doubt, if cigarette smokers *also smoked marijuana regularly*, their incidence of Lung Cancer was less than it should have been or would have been – without the marijuana. Marijuana Protects the Lungs even for Tobacco Smokers! The reduction in lung cancer for Marijuana smokers was statistically significant. The well-known researcher, Donald Tashkin stated in no uncertain terms:

"Carcinogenic Tars of Tobacco are De-activated by Smoking Marijuana" (Tashkin)

Prior to this research, in 2006 Tashkin carried out the largest study of its kind with 65,000 patients. It was conducted at the prestigious Kaiser Permanente, CA. Cancer patients were matched with a non-cancerous Control Group. Risk factors were compared. Tashkin reported that for Marijuana smokers there was **no** **"increased risk of lung cancer or other typically-tobacco-related-cancers."** Findings were consistent for different measures of Cannabis, such as *current, former and frequency of use.*

For Marijuana smokers of 10 to 20 years duration, the **risk was about one-third of non-users;** the magnitude of reduced risk was more pronounced for those who began Marijuana after age 20. Authors concluded:

> *Study suggests that moderate marijuana use is associated with reduced risk of squamous cell carcinoma of head and neck.* They noted that *experimental data have shown that cannabinoids inhibit cancer growth.*

Marijuana ~ To Avoid Lung Cancer.
More Important
For All Cigarette Smokers:
Marijuana ~ To Save Your Life!

In the pre-stage of lung cancer, the lungs are stagnant and without the necessary motility for health. Capacity is shrunken owing to non-use since the habit of the breath is shallow and small. If nicotine poisoning is added, the scenario can become life-threatening. Cells contract immediately to get away from the poison. Elimination and purification are retarded. Stagnation sets in as the addict injects tobacco smoke into the lungs usually at least once an hour which insures an increase in suffocation.

Marijuana Opposite to Nicotine:
As soon as Marijuana smoke enters the blood, there is a tremendous expansion of the sacs in the lung. If there was characterological constraint in the first place (and there probably was), there is correspondingly significant release of the constriction. This is the exact opposite of the nicotine effect. As the alveoli of the lungs expand, so does lung capacity. In addition, chest muscles relax so there is more room for expansion of the lungs. All in all, the *Marijuana Experience* is relief from the usual inhibition of the breath. Tension that breeds illness evaporates. The feeling is registered as "well-being," which may be part of the cure according to the IOM.

Oddly enough the high feeling of being relieved from stress is feared by the ignorant. To breathe fully, think clearly, feel happy and be healthy does not fit the conditioned agenda. But it is the remedy out of the Cancer Biopathy. Without the stress in the body, the breath deepens and becomes big - which re-ignites the natural balance.

With Marijuana:
Tars of Nicotine Do Not Lodge in the Lung.
Instead:
Efficient Lung Function Purifies and Oxygenates.

How much is inhaled is a direct response to how much has been exhaled. Increased inspiration is an automatic consequence to greater expiration.

Marijuana Facilitates Breathing:
The improvement in respiration that occurs with Marijuana has been known for thousands of years. In modern times, it is the reason that vast amounts of research and development have been conducted by the pharmaceutical giants in a quest to harness these benefits for diseases, such as lung cancer, emphysema and asthma – all of which are directly caused by an extreme inability to exhale. The hype concerning smoking of Marijuana as a cause of lung cancer via the tars produced in combustion has been thoroughly de-bunked by the government's own recent, broad-based research. Smoking is not what causes a problem for the lungs. Instead what is smoked determines the effects. That is not to say that the most efficient way to administer Marijuana is through a cigarette. Depending upon set, setting, preference as well as situation determines which route of administration will be best.

The specific bio-chemical benefits of Marijuana for lung cancer are multi-dimensional and have not yet all been envisioned and certainly not isolated and tested. In addition, some researchers have suggested that the multiple odor-producing molecules in the intact plant serve as protective:

> *Mercene* smells like mint and/or citrus. It is the most prevalent terpene in marijuana, known to be analgesic anti-inflammatory, anti-biotic and anti-carcinogenic. In aroma therapy, it is an anti-depressant. Mercene promotes THC effects. It interacts with the CBD cannabinoid and alters the permeability of the cell membrane, possibly allowing more THC to enter into the cell.

Limonene is another terpene abundant in cannabis resin. It has a strong citrus odor and is recognized as having anti-bacterial and anti-fungal qualities. Limonene inhibited a tumor-promoting gene in testing. With lung cancer studies, *Linomene* had anti-inflammatory effects on lung tissue exposed to tars. As an herbal, it is considered anti-depressant.

There is a whole host of odor producing molecules in Marijuana. They have been dismissed in the cancer studies with cannabinoids, since the mentality of the silver bullet cure-all rules. Terpenes in cannabis are considered defensive against plant predators and nothing more. None of their many possible synergistic protective actions are included in cancer research which portends a loss of efficiency in the long run.

> *It is not merely the monopoly of drug companies that causes concern ... danger of isolating so-called 'active' ingredients so that the modifying agents are left out ... may render the whole herb safe. These may not appear 'active' in isolated tests, but they offset side effects of active constituents.* (Bremness, World of Herbs)

Note:
This presentation is interested in the fundamental cause for disease without devolving into the many other instances that can lead to medical problems. Of course, it is a known fact that without the environmental toxicity of processed food, lungs (and for the matter all organs and regions of the body) could be less fertile ground for cancer. Inflammation would be less. Blood vessels would be more flexible, less sticky and further dilated. The modern diet is without question one of the major contributors to the expression of the Cancer Biopathy.

Review: Anti-Cancer Effects of Marijuana

1. Cancerous Tumors grow, thrive, travel and replicate, Marijuana stops the process. The tumor simply does not grow since DNA replication does not happen. It is stopped in the early stage of growth (*transcription*) Marijuana re-rights the confusion in bio-chemistry of the cell cycle. Tumors shrink rather than proliferate.

2. If deranged tissue has forgotten to self-destruct, studies demonstrate strong *apoptosis* (suicide response) if Marijuana is administered. The program for suicide becomes operational where it had been lost.

3. In addition, spreading (Metastasis) and over-growing the host does not happen if the cancerous tumor is treated with Marijuana. *Metastasis* has been proven to be rendered defunct as the response to cannabinoids.

4. And the *tumor shrinks* if injected with THC (from Marijuana). Shrinkage begins immediately.

5. The *Immune Response* is restored to competency with Marijuana. The organism wards off cancer cells.

6. The repercussions of chronic inflammation show clearly that chronic chaotic cellular over-activity seeds the ground for cancer. The anti-inflammatory action of Marijuana Therapy relaxes, resettles and balances the chemistry of the deprived tissue by re-nourishing the suffocating *areas of unconsciousness.*

Anti Cancerous Marijuana Effects Continued:

#7 Anti- Angiogenesis:
Starvation by Marijuana

Conservation of the body is served by constant replication of trillions of cells fulfilling specific functions; then disintegrating. But cancer cells have seceded from this holistic operation. They have a life of their own. Their goal is to reproduce, travel and settle down and take root in hospitable areas. Cancerous tissue needs nourishment to grow and divide and begin the process all over again. *Angiogenesis* is the growth of a bridge of blood vessels from healthy tissue to the tumor.

Marijuana stops Angiogenesis, That is: the tumor starves without nutrients and oxygen. According to the research, both CB1 and CB2 Receptors take part in a cooperative dual action of ridding the tumor of its mainline. There is *molecular cross-talk* among CB1 and the CB2 Receptor. That has been documented, but so far is not deciphered. Nevertheless, that the connectivity between the two receptors increases with Marijuana Therapy is known and its result is to restore Anti-Angiogenesis. It is not surprising that as the evidence mounts for Marijuana as a viable therapy for cancer, progressive Health Care Practitioners are coming forward in support:

> *cannabinoids found in marijuana may have a primary role in cancer treatment and prevention. A number of studies have shown that these compounds can **inhibit tumor growth.** In part, this is achieved by inhibiting Angiogenesis, the formation of new blood vessels that tumors need in order to grow.* (7/23/2001, Dr. Andrew Weil)

However, generally speaking, the communities of medicine, media and politics ignore the studies and the people are uninformed. To recognize that Marijuana is beneficial for treating and even preventing cancer is still not politically correct. Even though the National Cancer Institute has finally (2011), publicly but ever-so-quietly added Marijuana Therapy to its treatment protocol, suggesting that oncologists prescribe it as a sleep aide; an appetite enhancer; for pain **and** for its *anti-tumor properties*, this capitulation by the U.S. Government agency was not First Page news. Mega Industry monopolizes "breaking news" segments.

To date thousands of studies have proven the absolute safety of Marijuana and/or its natural compounds. Hundreds of scientific papers with strict protocol point unmistakably to the advantages of utilizing the phyto-chemicals of Marijuana in dealing with the Cancer Biopathy. Specific results confirm that THC inhibits formation of blood cells that feed the tumour. Tumour development is stopped as well as its spread! In addition, THC assists biochemical pathway (Autophagy) whereby deranged cells digest themselves.

Angiogenesis, Apoptosis, and Autophagy are bio-chemical safe-guards that become disordered in Cancer. They are demonstrably restored by *Marijuana Therapy. Drug Companies are continuously* attempting to exploit these results with patentable synthetic versions, while the *medical, scientific, political, judicial* mainstream blocks public knowledge of the relief for the cancer patient available from the whole plant:

"Further testing is needed" is the continuous litany.

Marijuana Therapy Intervenes in The Cancer Biopathy in All Processes Simultaneously and Efficiently to Restore Homeostasis

Speaking of Skin Cancer:
In holistic therapies, skin problems indicate breathing deficiency. The skin is the largest organ of respiration. It breathes. When it becomes clogged, it cannot fulfil its function of eliminating wastes. *Skin Cancer* can result. Since there are Cannabinoid Receptors all over the skin, scientists applied topical plant cannabinoids on areas of skin cancer. The Results: Plant cannabinoids stopped Angiogenesis to the cancer tissue and therefore stopped the progression of the cancer. This new evidence gives substance to *Oil of Cannabis* as in the *Holy Anointing Oil of the Bible* (Jeff Brown, Marijuana and The Bible); and the Indian Medical System, *Ayurveda* for prescribing *Oil of Bhang* to soothe skin 5000 years ago).

Marijuana is a Life-Saver:
Science is reversing its course and finally embracing the wisdom that came before. The kinship of the human being with Cannabis Sativa is obvious by subjective measure; objective observation of its effects; and by tests that detect invisible cellular activity. Many interesting facts concerning compounds of Marijuana and their effectiveness in skin cancer are known:

1. Both CB1 and CB2 Receptors are in abundance in the skin and are also present in cancerous skin tumours.
2. Skin Tumours show regression when Cannabinoid Receptors are activated via compounds of Marijuana.
3. Scientists have found at least two mechanisms for direct apoptosis of tumours.
4. Local administration of cannabinoids for treatment of non-melanoma skin cancer is being recognized as an alternative therapeutic for skin cancer.
5. Synergy between CB1 and CB2 Receptors elicits apoptosis. (http://www.jci.org/articles/view/16116)

Testimonials abound for Cannabis oils/salves from the intact plant that are curative and newsworthy but to date no serious research is planned to discover if the natural oils of Marijuana cure skin cancer. Instead and as usual, scientists continue to search for the *"attractive possibility of cannabinoid-based therapeutic strategies for skin disease/cancers (which is) devoid of non-desired CB_1-mediated psychotropic side-effects. (ibid)*

#8 Blood Velocity:
(Elimination / Purification)

One of the major functions of The Circulatory System is eliminating wastes. Its channels connect with the tiniest capillaries to clean the cells and also to wash away any cancerous tissue that may have been produced. Problems begin when the filtering system is plugged or its channels are narrowed by deposits or the flow is just too slow which allows for the buildup of noxious material causing problems, including and oftentimes: Cancer.

Marijuana Therapy immediately increases the fueling capacity of the lungs because of the immense expansion in both the oxygen gathering alveoli as well as the release of tension in the oppositional chest muscles that constrain and restrain the depth of the breath. There is simply more oxygen for transport. And there is more channel-width for transport because blood vessels dilate by the *Marijuana Effect*. This translates as less resistance in the vessels which results in systemic enhancement of the Circulatory System. Blood Velocity enhancement with Marijuana has been researched and verified in studies on the brain that were focused on the consciousness-raising features of the Cannabis Sativa plant and any interface with CB1 Receptor activation. (not addressed in this presentation)

92

Marijuana has a very unique effect on the organism. It enhances the oppositional mechanism of fluid balance of the organism as mediated by The Cannabinoid System. Marijuana is itself a dual acting agent which is cause for its synchrony with the body network. Since it produces simultaneous stimulation / relaxation, it is homeopathic in its individualized outcome. Marijuana Therapy is Holistic Medicine since it affects the entire organism, at once as an uplifting experience.

By increasing the velocity of the blood, *The Marijuana Effect* serves as medium of cleansing, filtration and purification. Not only are all channels enlarged and therefore more waste is removed at any one time, in addition, there is also faster streaming of discarding the entrenched toxins because there is a slight increase in heart rate. The river of waste therefore is moving just a tad faster and transporting its toxins out from the organism with greater speed. As an additional health benefit, there is a bit more of the more richly oxygenated nourishment (as per *The Marijuana Breath*) reaching into the cellular matrix. The result is that *cleansing, maintenance* and *nourishing* are enhanced.

Stagnation is eliminated through greater aeration in all areas. One could make a case here for the psychological component of increased blood velocity as it facilitates the cognition, creativity and even compassion of an individual life. (Not within this presentation.)

(Debunking The MYTH)

Marijuana Damages the Immune System.
FACT: Nothing Could Be Further from the Truth!

In keeping with the bifurcated operation in the organism for maintaining balance, The Immune System proceeds by a dual oppositional process. Just as stimulation and relaxation vacillate constantly throughout the organism in a flexible and dynamic balance, so does the healthy Immune System act against danger. One stroke of the immune response is aggressive: to fight / attack / ward off any foreign invasion perceived as threatening to the organism. In a brilliant system of checks and balances, the other polarity is an antithesis of the attacking mode. It *tones down* the reaction. **You can't have one without the other.** Health is the maintenance of balance. If the aggressive act is not **toned down**, the person will be destroyed (from within). If the calming mode is not offset by vigilance, the system will be asleep on the job - and the person will be destroyed (from without).

We imagine the dualistic properties of the Immune System as representing two opposite sides, but actually there is an intertwined unity. The healthy organism is all processes working in harmony to survive. Should a process become degraded or out of sync, the optimally functioning entity has myriad re-stabilizing structures and procedures that bend with the challenge. Medical problems develop when the excess stimulation or lethargy becomes chronic which signals failure of the equalizing pathways. This is the vicious circle of over-reactivity being over-compensated for by under-activity which is a self-propelling agenda that continues unless there is successful intervention. Analogy to the ups and downs of the see saw can be viewed as an example to show that those Immune Responses closest to the pivotal point of the pendulum are the healthiest. Movement is minimal at that position. Balance is easy to maintain.

In an overly-sensitized system, when a threat is perceived, too much immune response ranges from minor problems, as in simple allergies to a serious asthmatic attack. Conversely, immune reactivity may be insufficient as when cancer develops. Both extremes express habitual imbalance. Balance of the organism is designed so that when excitation is heralded because there is true danger, the extreme attacking mode of the immune response is **toned down** immediately and appropriately by the wisdom of the Modulating Principle of Health.

No Over-Reactivity - No Under-Reactivity
Cellular Expression of the Marijuana Life-Style

Dysfunctional Immune responses at either extreme are just different forms of Immune System Disease where the modulating principle is lost. In Multiple Sclerosis the attacking mode is unchecked while Cancer is over-stimulation that has progressed from slow, invisible suffocation to chronic inflammation (exhaustion of the immune response) and finally degrading to a lower life form that ferments rather than breathes.

The Holistic effect of Marijuana Therapy for a compromised Immune response cannot be denied. One of the main Cannabinoid Receptors (CB2) is found throughout the Immune System where it answers specific needs. Marijuana molecules impact it directly through the CB2 Receptor which is the customized linkage between Cannabinoid System instructions and Immune function which carries them out. Marijuana restores Immune Modulation by enhancement of regular breathing; through moderating extreme reactions; by relieving distress; by impacting Immune System cells to inhibit over-enthusiastic reactions to any potential, imagined or real danger.

"When inflammation goes off the handle, the body releases endo-cannabinoids ... that suppress the Immune System and takes down inflammation before it does more harm than good." (Melamede) That is, without the **toning down** of the immune response, there can easily be overpowering inflammation. Self-cells are attacked, organs degrade and death results.

The multi-tasking of Cannabis Sativa was deciphered by isolating effects of specific exogenous cannabinoids. It was found that there is definite, measurable **modulation** in autonomic processing with Marijuana administration. Over-reactivity which is symptomatic of imbalance is *toned down* by plant cannabinoids. An organism in tune with itself is definitive of health wherein the integrative communication, regulated, moderated and modulated by The Cannabinoid System is at optimal functioning.

Marijuana facilitates this complicated process from which the simple state of homeostasis results. If there is energetic lacking, the homeostatic process can go awry. Without the modulating principle in charge at this subtle level of immune reactivity, Cancer can be conceived. In other words, if respiration at the cellular level is subdued causing over-reactivity, inflammation and blockage (in that order), the originating cause of cancer exists. The cells are clogged. There is obstruction in the natural cycle of nourishment and elimination. It may be a small deficit in the operation of the major functions of the organism, but it is constant. Rather than oxygenation, there is putrification and fermentation. The Immune System is overwhelmed. It has lost the ability to defend the body through the dual processes of **toning down** the inflammation and at the same time, rejecting any unwelcome invasion. Marijuana Therapy rescues the exhausted Cannabinoid System. It reawakens its modus operandi of maintaining perspective, which in turn resets the myriad, complex cellular biochemical secondary operations of balance.

The Marijuana Effect of re-oxygenating the organism is primary from which all the cellular intricacies that have been enumerated become once again in line with the *Prime Directive of Survival of The Whole.*

#*10 Stress:*
(Mental Posture is Altered)

Marijuana as Reliever of Distress:
That intuitive knowledge espoused throughout ancient Indian texts is proven by modern science. Nevertheless, the primal magnetic enthusiasm between *marijuana molecules* and Cannabinoid Receptors is still not fully understood or appreciated. The increase in cellular vitality that occurs with Marijuana administering is clear under the microscope but no extrapolation to whole person health has taken place. While Marijuana has subjective and objective benefits for health, happiness, cognition and creativity; and oftentimes imparts a sense of unity, liberation and well-being, which although not lasting is also not forgettable, the extent that these states of being are opposite to the Stress Response is not understood nor is its significance realized.

Marijuana is Anti-Stress
Stress is loss of balance in the physical, mental and energetic matrix which advances from distortion in the *pattern of the breath* and which has been shown to be rehabilitated by *The Marijuana Breath.* Not only does our manner of breathing determine our experience but by altering it, we change our perceptions, attitudes, degree of health and level of consciousness. Although it surely is possible to change the insufficient habit of breathing through Breath Work Programs now easily accessible, such discipline requires time, will, knowledge, money and a continuous commitment to all those requirements, whereas the benefits of Marijuana are immediate, consistent, far-reaching, easily available, natural and proven.

In cases of Breast Cancer, statistics show that the disease is unquestionably influenced *by psycho-social factors and coping styles*. There is definitive proof that for breast cancer patients, the outlook is more positive if the patient has inner strength and is up to the challenge. The best prognosis is attached to a patient who has a sense of personal control / autonomy / and is not emotionally repressed. *The Marijuana Experience* is relaxation by oxygenation and diminishment of stagnation. The person is able to have a more global perspective and can take stock of everything since mental confusion dissipates with adequate breathing. Feeling competent and in charge of oneself is reflective of sufficiency in the breath.

Stress dysregulates the Immune System, setting up an unhealthy situation for everyone, especially those with cancer. When relaxation and forward thinking are out of reach, there is suppression of cell-mediated immunity: the primary defense against metastasis. Five thousand years ago, Chinese QIGONG masters taught the practice of breathing as the foundation of health and awareness. Each breath can bring more oxygen into the organism to stimulate vital organs and create a joyful calm that penetrates throughout the being, similar to a feeling of well-being or what is called *the high.*

(Anxiety originates from *to strangle,* which sheds light on the wisdom of the past. Limited breath gives rise to feeling anxious, a fact pretty much lost even to health care professionals today.)

> *Marijuana appears to promote development of new brain cells, has anti-anxiety and anti-depressant effects... other illegal and **legal** drugs have been shown to suppress the formation of new brain cells. Marijuana spurs formation of new brain cells in the hippocampus which reduces anxiety and depression.* (Zhang et al)

The study and especially the conclusions by Zhang et al, shamefully stands out because very few, if any other research team, have been willing to interpret Marijuana data with such objectivity, logic and honesty.

The conclusions continue:

> *Marijuana is the only illicit drug to produce increase in neurons...positively correlated with its (anti-anxiety) and anti-depressant-like effects.*

Zhang told United Press International **"a high dose of smoked marijuana, might also have the same effect"** but he is "not certain how many equivalent joints it would take." **Our results indicate cannabinoids could be used for the treatment of anxiety and depression!"** (and) **"marijuana should be used as alcohol or nicotine (and)** has been used for various diseases for years in other countries." (University of Saskatchewan)

Laughing ~ Breathing Correlation:
Many years ago, Norman Cousins reported curing his cancer with comedy (*The Three Stooges*). But rather than laughing himself better as he reported, in fact, laughing caused him to breathe without restraint. In fact, **he breathed himself better.** He no longer was burdened with his adult concerns, but gave himself over to a more youthful consciousness.

The *Marijuana Experience,* in its anti-stress mode is reminiscent of the childhood state of non-worry that is simply the result of the natural, non-inhibited breath accompanied by an optimally functioning Cannabinoid System. That **Good Mood consciousness,"** of the IOM is a rare release of tension experienced as a fuller than usual relaxation. The organism has more energy since there is more accessible oxygen. The Cannabinoid System is rebalanced.

An Imaginary Scenario:
You are a cancer patient. You are nervous and worried. Perhaps you are taking weakening chemotherapy to eradicate the tumor or undergoing surgery or worse. Maybe you are in pain, in discomfort, nauseous and without appetite. The path to healing is obviously not to remain in such a constricted state. To relax, breathe deeply and have an optimistic yet accepting attitude is unquestionably the healthiest mode to adopt. Being realistic, however, a cancer diagnosis brings fear. In addition, chronic characterological anxiety is not easily dissolved. Tranquilizers and anti-depressants are counter productive and just mask the reality. Neither can you will yourself to breathe and/or think properly! There are debilitating treatments, mental and physical exhaustion and sense of hopelessness lurking in the background.

Destroying the tumor will not solve the problem. The modern method of killing cancerous cells is just a stop gap. Revision of the tendency toward suffocation and relapse is the only sensible objective. Rarely (if ever) is it included in the treatment plan. As noted, today there are many progressive programs available for health conscious patients. Breathing Practices, Meditation, Non-toxic Diet, Stretching and Aerobic Exercise, Creative Work and wholesome entertainment are healing activities to be encouraged and incorporated into daily routines.

A certain intentional awareness is needed to succeed, along with regularity and constancy absolutely devoid of the striving mode of anxiety and shallow breathing. All these specifics without question aid toward recuperation of the whole person. To breathe freely and therefore to invite relaxation, positivism and acceptance, with no fear is the ultimate prescription for health evidenced in mental peace and mirrored in balanced autonomic processes. Such a favorable state is very far from realistic for the Cancer patient unless there is a life-altering about-face from what has been.

Marijuana Therapy serves as the *intervention* that can alter continuance of disease. Since Marijuana releases inhibited respiration, inhalation is deeper, exhalation is greater. That is, there is more and better fuel with less resistance in the form of toxins and stress. The tension of shallow rapid ineffective breathing gives way to the relaxation mode. Breathing returns to its natural responsibility of nourishing and cleansing the organism.

Marijuana Therapy facilitates autonomic balance. It **tones down** both physical and mental over-reactivity. Thoughts are unhurried and even suspended allowing for healing energies to emerge. In such a state there is receptivity which then invites acceptance. Indeed since marijuana is stimulant simultaneous with its relaxant effects, energy is increased and depression is lifted. Marijuana relieves pain, eliminates nausea, sparks appetite, aids sleep and facilitates digestion, easily responsible for a **"good mood consciousness,"** which encourages and makes achievable an intentionality or focused awareness that is impossible with tension.

It's All in the Breath is an ancient Indian proverb that holds great import for our modern world of excess and lost wisdom. Not only have we forgotten how to enhance the breath to relieve distress, there is not even any recognition that the way we breathe day in and day out definitely affects health and happiness; or that sustained increased energy transforms the personality to a higher state of being without stress.

Marijuana is a Facilitator of *The Breathing Process*.

Consciousness by Marijuana Therapy:
Health from the Healing Energies

Evolution with Marijuana:
Medicine and Philosophy were integrated disciplines through most of the 10,000 years of human records. Modern technology has severed the link between these two fundamentally interconnected areas of study. This section deals with higher order biological processes through which Marijuana impacts the human organism and **mandates that Science and Philosophy re-*merge*.** The *cause, effect, functions and direction* revealed by Retrograde Signaling is not understandable to the technological mindset. Whereas science is witness to the concrete operations by which the optimally functioning Cannabinoid System predicts what is needed before it is demanded and also **tones down** the potential strength of the demand before it occurs, no interpretation of these processes are forthcoming. The evidence that Marijuana Therapy not only rejuvenates this essential intuitive Mechanism of Balance but enhances its performance has meaning far beyond the ending of sickness.

Marijuana Upgrades the Retrograde Program To the Next Level of Competence.

The Cancer Biopathy impedes communication among the cells. The integrated sequential biological safeguards against over-reactivity are lost. Instead of order, there is disorder. Instead of relaxation, there is excitation with increased motility of cancerous cells wherein growth is uncontrolled. Cancerous tissue proliferates and spreads. If at this point in the Disease Syndrome, Marijuana Therapy is interjected into the mix, the frantic confusion at the molecular level is reversed and calm is restored. The Cancerous invasiveness is stopped. Tumors shrink. The deficient Cannabinoid System is not only reset; its functioning is actually enhanced by embracing the compounds of Marijuana.

Within the cellular matrix, the retrograde mechanism is reinstated. There is a slowing in signal transduction Over-reactivity is modulated and **toned down**. The organism is relieved of distress. What becomes visible under the microscope is experienced subjectively. It becomes clear that objective science and empirical understanding are just different aspects of the same identity. Just as there are (visible) intervals between molecular messages (in the body) there are (empirical) spaces between thoughts (in the mind). The *subjective* mental registration of time slowing down in the mental field simply reflects the unhurried (objectively observed) mode within the cellular matrix. It has been well documented that Marijuana Therapy invites the *Alpha State* of brain relaxation and receptivity. The competitive insecure anxiety is replaced by a *sense of well-being*. Breathing is easy, deep and regular. Self-centeredness evaporates; calm has replaced confusion in the cells as well as in the mind. The Cancer Biopathy cannot engage in such a set and setting! Such a state has recently and aptly been called: The Marijuana Lifestyle!

With Marijuana Therapy, Thinking is Slowed.
The Perennial Backdrop of Finer Energies Emerge.
Less **Signaling IS** *More* **Awareness**.

The Quiet Mind is Healing:
Thinking obscures Higher Consciousness. In this framework: *thinking as an obstacle to (Higher) consciousness or greater awareness speaks to non-essential clutter in the energetic field that imagines, worries, pretends, judges and rationalizes,* unrelated to planning, intuitive realizations, discrimination, creativity or study. The visible confusion in cellular operations is but the invisible counterpart of the continuous prattle that occurs most of the time in most people and which disallows finer, healing energies from emerging.

Whereas witnessing order in molecular processes is evident to the trained eye, watching the antics of one's own mind is tedious, requiring both will and skill. A restless mind is always too busy to notice its own continuous background of distraction. Psychological activity is of a finer energy than the material; thoughts are fast and uncontainable. But today thinking can actually be measured with technology. Excessive prattle translates as imbalance and subjectively registers as general anxiety or lack of ease evidenced by irregularity in the pattern of the breath and incongruence of brain waves. That is, thinking is lack of ease.

A Meditative State of Mind is Evoked by Marijuana As Demonstrated by the Slowness of Brain Waves.

Marijuana Affects Thinking:

Studies that have long-since been forgotten (1970's) proved that *The Marijuana Effect is accompanied by a slowing down of the frames that pass by in the mental sphere thereby allowing for greater focus to be expended on each frame.* (Sugarman & Tarter)

In that calm state, thinking is diminished. Tension is relieved. Energy is released and is therefore available to those areas of unconsciousness suffering from low levels of oxygenation (inattentiveness). Simultaneous to the physical benefits, there is subjective recognition of an energized serenity of (more) awareness, noticeably different from before Marijuana imparted its effects. There is an *alteration in the mind field which is termed Higher Consciousness.* Such an energetic state cannot be observed by the intellect because it takes place outside and beyond the realm of ordinary language and thought since it is of a finer energy.

While words are less than adequate to describe the *high*, nevertheless the momentary pause in thought (*and in cell activity*) is realized and appreciated subjectively as liberation from self worry or a feeling of well-being. *The High of Expanded Awareness* is an energetic in-pouring into the interval between thoughts **and** into the spaces between (cellular) messages. And the high heals! Evolution toward conscious action is seen in observable cellular cooperation as well as in the experiential mental harmony of Marijuana Therapy. For those suffering from the Cancer Biopathy, ***The Benefits of Marijuana can be understood as altering the energetic dissonance of grave imbalance to a finer than usual state of resonance*** evidenced by science and supported by millions who welcome ***The Marijuana Experience.***

IT GIVES PAUSE

Higher Consciousness:
It is no coincidence that with the advancement of materialism, consciousness has become denigrated while the incidence of systemic illness has increased. We are beings in need of time for solitude, silence and serenity. But modern living is constant socialization, stimulation, noise, confusion and competition. To disengage from worldly conditioning, at least to some intentional extent, is a mandate for superior health, since the cultural goals of productivity and performance are opposed to independent thought. Constant challenge and continuous entertainment cause loss of balance which is responsible for the neurotic personality. Marijuana Therapy provides the dysregulated Cannabinoid System the welcomed opportunity to regain its *modulating, moderating and regulating* function, simultaneously remaining in the fray but without the fervor of fear of failing. Deep breathing indicates *dis*-identifying with the confusion even in the midst of turmoil. An inner sense of lost familiar composure returns.

Rather than succumbing or adding to the imbalance of any situation, the individual who is rehabilitated with Marijuana Therapy stands above/outside the disorder. This ability to distance oneself psychologically from whatever is non-essential and chaotic is inherently connected to the physiological relaxation of the Marijuana Experience as documented by science. It is also that serene state of conscious observing that is feared by those who are identified with cultural goals rather than universal values.

Feeling LOW Preferred: *(by the Dominant Culture)!*
In an incredible, ironic, unfortunate yet understandable state of human affairs, generalized tension throughout the population and **not** relaxation serves the status quo. Tension insures dependency on the system, thereby setting the agenda for citizens to be more easily molded, while *Higher Consciousness* is inherently feared since it awakens interest in essential values which stand against the superficiality of the status quo.

In an osmotic twist of philosophical concurrence, the healing professions and the scientific community are aligned with the ambitions of the materialistic culture. Despite the reality that *feeling good* and/or *feeling high* is unquestionably more in keeping with regaining health than *feeling bad* or *feeling low*, there is a deep-seated aversion to natural, holistic, time-worn techniques for health since both profit and authority are lost to the professional. Patients in a *good mood consciousness* rather than in a bad mood are less likely to be dependent on the doctor or the priest.

There are Spaces between Thoughts
As there are Intervals between Cellular Signals.

It is only when the mind is completely at rest without any distraction that the spiritual realm of the healing, finer energies can be received which is why all practices geared toward self-development aim for curtailing thought. Biofeedback, yoga, karate, running, meditation, tai chi, prayer, chanting, breath-work are all popular paths to relieving stress, regaining balance and quieting the mind. It is no accident that Marijuana was employed in the esoteric disciplines. It was intuitively recognized as a facilitator for serenity and bliss.

Today just the sheer number of different methods to still the mind, center the focus, afford relaxation, give one a sense of peace, security and competence are indicative of the collective confusion. The imbalance of daily living is far removed from (the perceived) carefree security of childhood before balance was lost and breathing was full. The adults of the world have become destabilized and the children will soon follow. Desire and competition are overwhelming. Wanting more and getting more and wanting more and getting sick is the story of the modern society. There is no place for relaxation, no space for solitude. Stress is the name of the game. And the ultimate consequence of playing is too often the Cancer Biopathy.

In Summary:
Marijuana Therapy offers a Higher Consciousness, described as a *good mood, sense of security,* feeling of *wellness* and even an experience of *ecstasy.* Regardless of the terms, it speaks to a global rather than self-centered mentality. Healing is natural and founded in the biology of calm (silence). None of these descriptions is appreciated or embraced by the medical mentality. Objective science does not acknowledge that the physical reality, proven under its own microscopes, has profound meaning within human subjective experience. What is felt by the person with Marijuana is an uplifting mood, best explained with mystical adjectives.

Regardless of any individualized account, there is undeniable, observable magnetism of the body for the *Healing Molecules of Marijuana* and consequential, predictable alteration of the mind toward a deeper awareness that is not understood, appreciated or accepted. Instead it is seen as a threat!

Society fears fundamental questioning...represses it (as) dangerous...it could spread a contagion of doubt (and) undermine blind loyalty to social authority.
(Ernest Becker)

Mainstream Medicine wants to eliminate the uplifting experience. *Altered consciousness* is restoration to finer energy levels lost along the struggle of existence. By seeking to eradicate the *high* perspective, Western Science has missed the point of holistic remediation. To shun so-called "psychotropic" effects that function through The Cannabinoid System, the pharmaceutical complex rejects the proven healing that accompanies **toning down** reactivity through natural balancing and without one directional dangerous drugs. Whether the opposition to Marijuana stems from fear of loss of control or loss of money, it is clear that derision directed at the ancient plant is irrational, unscientific and self-serving. By remediation of Marijuana Therapy, instead of impulsive, often inappropriate actions, there is an immediate, observable *inhibition of irrelevant signaling.*

In contrast to living the harried (internal) lifestyle that is fertile ground for cancer, there can be balance and healthy breathing so that relief from distress and even hints of more substantive realities interpose themselves occasionally. Such a state is available, accessible and enjoyed by millions of persons around the world who are regular partakers of the *good mood consciousness* that **is** *The Marijuana Experience* and which guides the subject through the stress of existence while affording health of body and mind where *one is in the world but not of it. (Krishnamurti)*

The Potential is in The Pause:
Healing Energies
Come through the Silence
Between Action

Consciousness
Comes through the Spaces
Between Thoughts

Marijuana Deepens the Silence
Slows the Action
Expands the Spaces

Hypothetical Subtle Benefit of Marijuana::

Higher Healing Energies:
Marijuana is a very complicated herb and one that undoubtedly will continue to be investigated. In the future even more will be understood concerning its seemingly limitless benefits for all things human. These are the early years of modern re-discovery during which time the ancient veneration of Marijuana has barely begun to be appreciated. The biological intricacies, historical controversies, the vast past uses of its medicinal applications, its former industrial global necessity, and including the higher perspective it may offer a society on the brink of extinction, are topics to be studied in the coming generations.

Future Appreciation of Marijuana:
Hypothetically speaking, the proven and extensive healing properties of Cannabis Sativa may be correlated with its super ability to absorb ultra violet light. Relevant areas to investigate:
1) Do the exogenous cannabinoids impart beneficial interactions in the cells owing to the incorporation of inordinately high levels of solar energy in the resinous flowers of Marijuana?

2) Do accompanying similar UV-B absorbent phyto-chemicals of the plant also upgrade the functioning of the organism by sharing their finer radiant energies?

3) Is there a primal (not yet imagined/examined) connection between these exceptionally protective molecules of the ancient Cannabis Sativa that withstand, absorb and incorporate solar energy, and the natural and gentle healing that results when the higher energy is merged with the human organism?

4) Finally: Is the *Marijuana Alteration in Consciousness* nothing more than incorporating the measurably higher energetic charge of the molecules of Marijuana?

Relevant Scientific Facts:

THC (and other cannabinoids) possesses **high UV-B absorption properties** *(280-315nm)* that are stored in the cannabinoid-rich trichomes (glands) on the plant surface and which may protect against predators while also shielding the seeds from ultraviolet rays. Hardly recognized as possessing health-imparting qualities are the terpenoids of delightful fragrance and the flavonoids of delicious taste prevalent on the surface of the fern-like leaves and ripening fruit of Marijuana that produce their own UV-B-absorbing compounds to protect the plant from otherwise killing rays.

Ultra violet light is a known carcinogenic and can cause mutations in DNA. Solar radiation is shielded by the atmospheric envelope. But that is changing. As we continue to damage the atmosphere, our race and other earth creatures are dying out slowly, imperceptibly, predictably and definitely. There is an ever-increasing amount of Ultra-violet-B rays that is endangering all life. Genetic mutations are evident in frogs, bats and people. The bees are disappearing. So are the birds. Body systems are over-run by a toxic environment. Even if we could breathe with natural efficiency, what we are breathing is becoming hazardous to our survival.

We Need A Miracle:
Cannabis Sativa Is It!

A wealth of scientific knowledge has surfaced. It cannot be ignored even though it is extremely inconvenient and politically incorrect. The ancient medicine that is so beneficial to the human organism is a natural remedy for rehabilitation of the planet; the air; the water; all sentient beings and the barbarism of the culture. Its agricultural name is *Hemp, and it has, of course, its own very amazing story that has been told many times. A unique but often overlooked feature is relevant here. It is a bit off topic,* but just for one paragraph:

The Very Good News:

Cannabis Sativa agriculture is responsible for producing enormous quantities of Biogenic Volatile Organic Compounds (BVOCs), called "mono-terpenes." They vaporize off the plants, rise into the atmosphere and reflect solar radiation away from the Earth. The vaporization seeds cloud formation which shields the planet's surface. BVOCs dissipate quickly. Theoretically, a constant stream of their vaporization is needed to protect the earth continuously. Fortunately, Cannabis grows all over the world and produces essential food at the same time that it produces an abundance of bio-fuels, therapeutics, building materials, biodegradable plastics and paper, cloth ... There really isn't any time left to argue. Every Spring that passes is an opportunity that is gone forever.

(http://www.physorg.com/news97214097.html)
General Science, *Biology,* May/2007

Protectiveness of Cannabinoids:
There is no doubt that the punishing limits of the human organism are being sorely tested. The forecast is that **Cancer** will be the **Number One Killer** in developed nations in a just a few short years. Inordinate amounts of ultra-violet-B are cause for trees being stunted; crops being more susceptible to pests; DNA damage and modification in gene expression. In general, plants die when under the overwhelming glare of ultra-violet-B light: **But not the Marijuana plant!** Instead it just oozes out more of its protective oils and absorbs as much sunlight as it possibly can. Cannabis is not structurally harmed with the UV-B radiation that is deadly to most other plants. None of its functions are restricted nor are there any changes in growth or vitality. The oils that the plants give off protect it completely!

As mentioned, certain Marijuana molecules are **patented by the U.S. government for their anti-inflammatory qualities**. Law states no patent will be awarded for a natural plant. To circumvent that logic, the government has patented specific benefits of the plant. There is yet more to the doubletalk. The government also has patented the "**Neuro-Protective features of Cannabis.**" Only those of us whose interests are basically *Marijuana-centered* are privy to the information about the *Preventive Secret Medicine* soon to be released to the misinformed public as a newly discovered patented invention being sponsored by the government or its agents. Plant cannabinoids stop pathological over-reactivity which leads to chronic inflammation and down the line more serious diseases, such as cancer. This is the "Anti-Inflammatory" effect of Cannabis patented by the government.

To Recount:
1) The Government Owns the *Anti-Inflammatory* benefits of marijuana which means that the government has the *right for exclusivity.*

2) *Neuro-Protective* features of these compounds are also patented by the government. It has at the same time in very definite language for many, many decades: that *Marijuana has no medicinal value.* The most sensitive and complicated specialized cells (*neurons*) of the body (comprising the entire nervous system) are responsible for movement as well as cognitive and life-sustaining processes. And these supremely important cells are protected by the cannabinoids that protect the plant. It is this basic and natural shielding and healing synergy between Marijuana molecules and the neurons of the body that has been seized by the U.S. Government Patent. That is, the anti-inflammatory and protective mysterious power of intact Marijuana cannot be used by anyone unless controlled by official government licensure / proclamation!

3) *Neurogenesis* - In its service to neuronal protection, there is strong evidence that the cannabinoids from marijuana have caused brain cells to grow! This startling information is offered in explanation for how Marijuana aids the organism in mental distress, such as its ability to lessen anxiety and **tone down** the episodes of bipolarity.

4) *Alzheimer's Progression Slowed*: Definitive studies prove that Marijuana Therapy helps to preserve the complicated cognitive connections of brain function. Scientists suggest this may explain the demonstrable Benefits of Marijuana Therapy for Alzheimer's. Suffice it to say that the upgrade in brain function that occurs with administration of Marijuana manifests in greater clarity, less confusion and less agitation. Therefore there is more relaxation, greater ability to think and more relaxation and steadiness of performance.

The closer to the sun, the greater is the content of THC. Studies from the 70s demonstrated a definite increase in THC in plants grown in high altitudes where there is a greater intensity of light and a greater amount of ultra violet rays in the spectrum.

The more ultra violet light that Cannabis Sativa is exposed to the more is the content of THC in the plant. Samples with the highest ratios (of delta-9-THC to CBN/CBD) came from regions whose sunshine was least attenuated by cloud cover, a variable affecting levels of UV-B irradiances. (Pate, 1979)

Note: Because of prohibition, much Marijuana is grown indoors without benefit of the sun. Yet very high potency Marijuana is grown even without UV-B radiation since plant heritage has been carefully selected and the strains represented are from high altitude areas with UV-B intense radiation. Just by its virtue of co-evolving with humans, Marijuana with the highest psychoactive properties is selected as of greatest value. Inside cultivating is a superb and innovative science driven by a determination to grow the best Marijuana regardless of obstacles. Nowadays progressive indoor growers utilize techniques that add appropriate levels of UV-B radiation.

The Philosophical Framework:
In Eastern cosmology, the sun is the finest energy manifest in this universe; as such, it is the highest *state of consciousness* or vibration to which an aspirant may attain. It is *enlightenment*. To transcend identification with the individual body/mind defines a person who realizes the Unity of all manifestation. There can be no question that *Anandamide* was named with forethought and knowledge. "Ananda" is an esoteric reference to pure cognition. It is the Bliss that is the goal of all mysticism. Identification with the individual body/mind is superseded by a universal and non-dual perspective, untainted by self-serving motives. No doubt, it is an aspiration for many but attainment of few. Nevertheless, The *Marijuana Experience* lends a momentary hiatus from the usual low level confusion so prevalent in human life to an experience aptly described as "high."

While ultra-violet rays are far too strong for direct human incorporation, encapsulation of that finest energy into a plant is natural, compatible and beneficial to all earth creatures. Plants are fed by the light of the sun. A tomato absorbs the spectrum of light compatible to its genotype. The fruit of the Marijuana plant does no less. It adapts, thrives and mercifully lends its natural radiant energy to receptive earth creatures.

More THC
Greater Spaces between Synapses
Longer More Frequent Pauses
Inviting
Healing Conscious Energies

Plant Cannabinoids Increase The Pause
Enlarge the Space
Expand the Possibilities
Enhance the Vibration

Classification of Marijuana Medicine:
There are many ways of classifying medicines. In the traditional sciences, a *supreme* medicine evokes balance: by moderating over-reactivity of the body; through modulating emotional extremes; by calming mental disturbance; and in imparting a higher level of functionality by reason of its inherent natural and complicated synergy with the system at hand. A Supreme Medicine is a *nourisher* of life and is effective in multiple disease syndromes, without distressing or damaging side effects. *It is tonic, adaptogenic and de-stressor all in one.* Such is the Supreme Marijuana Medicine. The Effectiveness of Marijuana Therapy is unquestionable except by those who deny science or misinterpret studies. It is a gentle, compatible remedy and its effects are cumulative.

The immediate relief that marijuana affords emanates from fuller breath which energizes, stabilizes and de-stresses and affords natural raising of consciousness. Only over time, however, with regular utilization of the plant is there long-term remediation in the pattern of the breath and the ensuing benefits. Just as the runner, the boxer, ballet dancer, yoga devotee and musician must always practice to maintain expertise in their craft, so must the Cancer patient maintain full and regular patterns in the breath all the time.

Long-Term and Regularly-Administered Marijuana Maintains Equilibrium by Deep, Rhythmic Breathing.

List of Holistic Benefits of Marijuana:
Marijuana Therapy is Not Toxic. It is Non-Invasive. Marijuana smoothes the processes of Aeration; Cooperation; Circulation, Communication; Elimination; Exhalation; Filtration; Inhalation; Inspiration; Moderation; Modulation; Oxygenation; Purification; Regeneration; Relaxation and Assimilation. In addition, Marijuana is Analgesic; Anti-Inflammatory; Anti-Emetic; Anti-Epileptic; Anti-Stagnating (disallowing fermentation); Bronchi-Dilating (against suffocation); Immune-Modulating Mood-Stabilizing; and Neuro-Protective. Incredibly this list is just a sample of the benefits of marijuana. But The Medical Model Bias persists: *Because of the Psychotropic Effects of some Cannabinoids, Clinical Use is Limited.*
http://www.biosignaling.com/content/8/1/12

Marijuana Therapy is a Botanical Medicine. It is safe precisely because it is prepared from the whole plant comprising both active and inactive phyto-chemicals that operate non-aggressively with a proven synergy. Cannabis Sativa is a Tonic-Herb which is mild in action, curative over time through gentling, nourishing and strengthening organs and systems toward rebalance. Marijuana as a Superior Remedy is an Instigator of the Healing Process by its Enhancement of The Breath.

Marijuana Attenuates the Imbalance of Cancer.
Equilibrium Dissolves the Cancer Syndrome.

Additional Information:

Rhabdomyosarcoma is a cancer that arises from skeletal muscle cells. (Science: "Rhabdomyosarcoma"). **THC lowered the viability of rhabdomyosarcoma cells.** According to basic research at the Complutense University of Spain, both synthetic cannabinoid, HU210 and natural THC decreased Rhabdomyosarcoma.

Science:
Risk of Head and Neck Cancer Reduced in Cannabis Users. In a large epidemiological study (a working group of scientists of several universities of the USA: Rhode Island, Massachusetts, Louisiana, and Minnesota) investigated the effects of Cannabis use on the development of a certain head and neck cancer (head and neck squamous cell carcinoma). Information of cannabis use by 434 patients was compared with data of 547 healthy subjects. After adjusting for potential other risk factors (i.e., tobacco smoking and alcohol drinking), Cannabis was associated with a statistically significant decrease of this cancer. **Risk was decreased 48%.**

Researchers at the University of New York: **THC inhibits cellular respiration of human oral cancer cells**. Scientists noted that "*results show cannabinoids are potent inhibitors of Tu183; are toxic to this highly malignant tumor.*" (Whyte DA, Pharmacology 2010)

The Endo-cannabinoid *Anandamide* **induces Cell Death in Colon Cancer.** (Int. J. Oncology 2010)

One person in three dies of cancer these days.

######
End Part III

PART 1V

Introduction

In the world of capitalism, it is only logical for the Pharmaceutical Industry to try to duplicate the *magic marijuana molecules*. The **Third** type of Cannabinoid is a molecular copy of (any number of) the phyto-chemicals of marijuana, synthesized in the laboratory so that it can be patented/controlled/prescribed for the purpose of profit as Natural Plant compounds cannot be!

Artificial manufacture of THC has actually been a licensed drug for decades, sold under the name Marinol, having first been designed to mimic the anti-nausea benefits of the whole plant. It is of course, just one of the 80 or so known interconnected cannabinoids of Marijuana. As such, it has not been even remotely as compatible or as merciful as nature. But by fabricating a facsimile of THC, Pharmaceutical Companies have overcome legal barriers to patented rights over a natural substance. In practice, the efficacy of just one of the over 500 compounds of Cannabis Sativa has proven to be a rather dismal failure, one fraught with the need for dosage, tolerance and even discomfort since it is no longer in its safe and gentle herbal form but has become a one-directional molecule with untested pitfalls.

The search continues and the rush is on to develop an artificial facsimile to tap into the balancing activity of **The Cannabinoid System** as a cure for the escalating chronic diseases of disharmony. It is a profit driven contradiction to have named an entire essential guiding component of earth creature-life after a very useful and famous plant while simultaneously slandering its most significant effect of a *feeling of well-being. (IOM*, 1999)

The Potential Disaster of Attempting to Intervene in the Complexity of Nature Cannot be Over-stated.

What is Cancer Research Looking For:
Something Far Better Than What It Has So Far!

Searching for What?
Billions of dollars on cancer research are spent every year. Scientists are tweaking the tails of different molecular compounds in laboratories around the world to produce a "new" magic drug that **stops cancer from growing, relieves the suffering, eases the unbearable side effects** of medical treatment and **does not harm** the physical or psychological integrity of the patient. If this sought after synthetic molecule could **prevent cancer** by removing its cause while also being a **healthy addition** to the patient's regular routine, the research would be miraculous and the scientists would be rich. From a higher perspective than the profit-motive, the number one criteria would be *Safety*, i.e. not toxic or addictive and already successfully tested on a varied human population over an appreciable length of time to assure no long-range limitation or danger. Second on the list of preference would be *no added discomfort* (physical or mental) whatsoever to the patient, but instead, a general easing of suffering. Custom-tailored choice of *comfortable delivery* depending upon patient need would be factored into the magic equation. In the real world, no discovery even approaching such high expectations has been manufactured.

Cancer Research is a Failure:
Years of research and billions of dollars later - no patentable drug fulfills the standards. **Chemo-therapy** is frightening, further degrading the patient's overall health that makes one so sick and weak that untimely death is too often welcomed.

(Marijuana was recognized first as an effective medicine for its amazing ability to control the unbearable nausea of traditional "chemo" allowing even the sickest patients to take nourishment.)

Radiation as the word connotes, is more lethal treatment. It is localized and more controlled than indiscriminate systemic poisoning. Treatment is never long-term. The patient either responds or dies. **Surgery** that cuts away the damaged and deranged tissue to halt its further spreading is rarely done without one of the other treatments (in less lethal dosage). Meanwhile the hunt continues. Science is searching out a cure without taking time to investigate cause. It wants any *drug, procedure or treatment that kills the cancerous tissue but not the patient.*

Whatever "Cure" is Discovered Must be Patentable:
Has to have a patent - otherwise no money to be made:
This imagined **magic bullet** must be new and not time-tested or natural. Otherwise no one profits. Patents produce money and spur motivation. Anything even suggestive of curing cancer that is *not patentable* is actually a threat to the pharmaceutical industry, and as such will predictably be disregarded and denigrated. *The greatest medical fairytale invention would be a substance, procedure, treatment or technique, proven safe over years for considerable types of cancers, in a wide assortment of circumstances and locales with ease of production, storage, and accessibility that is economically feasible and easy to administer that would: stop the cancer in its tracks; stop it from metastasizing; help the patient to feel better immediately; gently restore balance and health to the patient over time; and that prevented cancer in the first place throughout the general population.*

**The Benefits of Marijuana Fulfill
the Objectives of Cancer Research!
But Alas it Cannot be Patented!**

121

The Problem with the Marijuana Cure:
Even though studies demonstrate without a doubt that **Marijuana Cures Cancer** in the test tube, in animals and in human subjects, the incredible health *benefits of marijuana* serve only patients. Drug Companies can't make money on a plant! A doctor is hardly needed to prescribe or monitor totally safe vegetation that has been utilized in nearly all civilizations for health and well-being since the beginning of time. The entire TEN billion dollar governmental police/prison/legal complex becomes marginalized without its main artery of prohibition of Marijuana. Not only will all of the positions having to do with arrest, interdiction, adjudication, imprisonment and myriad accompanying industry slots become unnecessary when/if the widespread health benefits of the Marijuana plant become well-known and legally available, but if the public learns that **Marijuana really cures cancer**, what might happen to the health-care system, the pill manufacturers, urine-analysis agencies and Drug Programs? In reality, the danger to the capital-based, competitive structure is far greater than can be described in this work and encompasses all manner of societal restructuring and goals. Suffice it to say, that although many in the health care professions are privy to the truth about the healing effects of marijuana, none can ascribe to such a radical acceptance without stepping away from the establishment.

The Cannabis Doubletalk: (No Profits?)
"The profit system puts the pure cannabis herb at a disadvantage. Pharmaceutical Manufacturers are not going to put time and money into a substance they can't patent." (Woodsen) Predictably, there is a frantic race to pharmaceuticalize at least a piece / copy of the ancient, health-imparting natural phenomenon. The process of manufacturing tinctures, extracting from the plant by heating, juicing, freezing and vaporizing are all patentable (as noted) and considered *new procedures.*

Pills, potions, patches, lozenges, suppositories, salves and sprays are being invented and produced in the hope of cashing in on the new miracle DRUG to be extracted or synthesized from Cannabis Sativa.

The LIE of What's Wrong with the Intact Plant:
Of course, such a great effort to find something other than Marijuana to cure cancer or help so many chronic and debilitating diseases is not a sign of Drug Company compassion. Similarly, there is no acknowledging that the sole motivation for finding a cure for cancer is money. Instead two main lame reasons for not employing the intact plant are offered.

1) The "high" is part and parcel of the benefits of the Marijuana plant. Indeed, the Institute of Medicine stated that the "high" should be called a feeling of *well-being* or *good mood consciousness* and may be an inherent comforting and actually curative property of Marijuana. (How very right they are will be further discussed!) Notwithstanding this official position of the government funded study, the Drug Companies actually offer the subjective experience of **well-being or good mood** as the main reason another substance must be invented! Since they are continuously pointing out that at all costs, a good mood must be avoided. The search continues for a single, one directional molecule that masks, palliates the (symptoms of) cancer, or even cures it – without that stigmatized *feeling of "well being"* attached to it.

2) Standardization is used by the industry as another important reason to continue the search. It is, no doubt a meaningful requirement when "prescribing" a life-threatening unnatural substance that needs to be monitored for its safety and efficacy. But that is not the case with the beneficial and utterly safe flowers from the Cannabis Sativa plant. Rather the effects of Marijuana are not test-tube predictable and are instead dependent on the set and setting as well as the patient's own idiosyncrasies and individual state of health.

Beyond any doubt: the synergistic curative effects of marijuana *have been proven over and over again.* **Nevertheless, the benefits are incompatible with the medical / pharmaceutical complex.**

Studies with Marijuana Therapy Buried:
The evidence that intact Marijuana was a promising cancer cure was purposefully concealed by the United States Government. The study and the shameful story are profusely reported in cyberspace. There is even a Facebook Club in The Lie. A Breast Cancer Study in 1974 found very positive results with administration of Marijuana. It was stunningly clear that the compounds in Marijuana stopped the cancerous tissue from spreading. Indeed, as we now have seen, when cannabinoids are injected into malignant tumors – the tumors shrink, which is exactly what happened in 1974. The results were simply shelved and the research was erased from public knowledge. Of course, further studies in the Dark Ages of the truth about Marijuana in the U.S. were banned. Prohibition reigned.

Thankfully on the international scene, research moved forward and continued to demonstrate great benefits for cancer treatments from Marijuana. What happened in 1974 could not happen today. (Let's hope) The truth can no longer be kept from the public. It is available in the atmosphere to all who can google! Although for the most part, the mainstream media in the U.S. maintains the code of silence concerning the dramatic and magnificent health-imparting wonders of Marijuana, the unyielding determination of patients, activists and some noble scientists, altogether has persevered. **The effects of Marijuana on the cancer syndrome are absolutely clear:** Marijuana shrinks breast and brain cancer and limits prostate cancer. When smoked, the results have quite surprisingly pointed to protection from lung cancer. (Details presented in the following pages.)

The question remains: Why do doctors keep saying: *"That does not mean you should start smoking marijuana to prevent and cure cancer?* The logical response to such blatant disregard of scientific evidence is **Why NOT?**

As reported under the Brain Cancer section of this presentation, the most recent report to uphold the benefits of natural cannabinoids specific to Brain Cancer recounts unprecedented and unexpected shrinkage of a tumor over a period of years owing to daily marijuana smoking by two teenagers. This was not a clinical study with a control group because, although Marijuana is used by millions of teenagers and young adults around the world on a regular basis, the Medical Profession and Pharmaceutical Industry are both afraid of the side effects of the natural plant on real people.

The study was well-documented and reported by professional scientists. It followed appropriate protocol over the six year follow-up of two teenage girls. In both cases, the brain cancer tumors quite mysteriously just kept shrinking over the course of being monitored on a regular basis. In both cases, the cancerous tumors could not be fully excised during surgery. The prognosis for both patients was guarded and certainly there was no expectation of the tumors dissolving. Only as the patients continued toward full recovery did they admit their illegal and regular use of marijuana, fittingly called *The Marijuana Lifestyle*. (March, 2011)

To date no further such studies are planned by the Medical Profession or the Scientific Community.

Note: In all the literature, I found only one doctor who stepped out of the mainstream box. In his study of marijuana and brain cells, **Dr. Zhang** said "marijuana appears "to be the only illicit drug whose capacity to produce increased...neurons is positively correlated with its (anti-anxiety) and anti-depressant-like effects."

In the study, a synthetic cannabinoid copied from Marijuana was injected into rats for ten days which according to Zhang was the equivalent of a "high dose" of smoked marijuana, without being able to say how many joints it would equal. Even though the synthetic was injected, Zhang acknowledged that *there would not be a difference if enough marijuana were smoked.* This study was not about cancer, but demonstrated that marijuana caused new brain cells to grow which Zhang believed might be one of the reasons that marijuana reduces anxiety and depression. Hopefully the courage of this researcher will be followed by other scientists who are interested in exposing the truth.

Marijuana Therapy which allows calm in the face of the storm, relaxation regardless of external hostilities so that one is able to function smoothly and to maintain equanimity in the midst of a disharmonious atmosphere is the safest, efficient remedy for the modern discord of which The Cancer Biopathy is the most widespread and feared expression. This *ancient herb of renown* restores the organism to equilibrium gently and efficiently with ease and *reliability. It re-invigorates the ebbing life force to the level of self-healing so as to disengage the rampant decaying of the body that takes place with Cancer.* Marijuana Therapy is not an attack on the expression of the disease but simply aids the functionality of the *burnt out* Cannabinoid Network.

Head and Neck Cancer Study:
"Maybe you *could* smoke enough!"

Recent documentation of the preventive benefits of Marijuana was conducted to determine what effect, if any, marijuana might have on Head and Neck Cancers. This was a longitudinal study without clinical aspects that looked into the lifestyles of groups of people:

Marijuana smokers of 20 year duration were compared to non-smokers during the same 20 years. Included were people under 60 who had smoked at least 11 marijuana cigarettes a day for 20 years. The control group was comprised of citizens in the same age range who did not use marijuana. Again, the results are stunning!

Front page feature was deserved and predictably denied. Only those who search out the findings on the internet know the reality: There was a 46% diminished incidence of Head and Neck Cancers (throat, esophagus, tongue and brain) in the group who smoked Marijuana (heavily and regularly) for over 20 years! This statistic is in tune with those marijuana smokers who were protected from developing lung cancer even though they smoked tobacco; with the reduction in breast cancer tumors by 50%; and for the favorable findings of marijuana with Prostate Cancer; Lymphoma and Bone Cancer.

The point is simple and revoltingly redundant for all studies: Marijuana Palliates the Symptoms of Cancer; Diminishes the Rate of Cancer; Decreases Expression of The Cancer Biopathy; Stops the Spread of Cancer – all the while imparting a positive outlook on life, now known as simply *a good mood consciousness*. Could it really be so? To reduce your chances of the dreaded diagnosis of cancer by 50%, Marijuana Therapy over the course of a lifetime is recommended?

Long Term Heavy Marijuana Smoking
Diminishes Head/Neck Cancer.

Capitalism and Government Against People:
The Laws are changing but the Propaganda Remains. Pharmaceutical Companies continue extraction, juicing, copying, vaporizing, etc. to produce a distorted and diminished form of Marijuana that can be patented and sold - **without that dangerous feeling of well-being**. In a capitalistic world, this makes sense. Companies exist to make money! Whereas the U.S. Government exists to serve the public, its alignment with the profits of pharmaceutical companies has disregarded its prime directive of service to the people, thereby depriving citizens of a medicine that is timeless.

As we have seen, Marijuana restores the organism to cooperative functioning. Damaged cells are discarded. No further metastatic contamination occurs. The Cancer Biopathy is rendered Defunct.

The Holistic Effect of Marijuana:
This release of tension that occurs with Marijuana Therapy is a result of innumerable, incredibly complex, bio-chemical cooperative processes of the nearly 500 compounds of Cannabis Sativa flowers that balance and enhance the metabolic pathways of the organism and in no way can be even infinitesimally approximated by a one directional artificial molecule.

In traditional medical wisdom, oxygen is understood as gross fuel for the body, nevertheless there is more to "livingness" than just breathing in oxygen. In this very same way, there is more to the Benefits of Marijuana than just one or two cannabinoids. There is a synergy, a synchrony, a symphony that comes from a rhythmic, easy, deep slow and quiet way of receiving that energy.

Interesting Notes of Irony

There are now more than 10,000 cannabinoid citations in PubMed. To date, there are **over 20,000 published studies or reviews** in the scientific literature pertaining to marijuana and its active compounds. That total includes over 2,700 separate papers published on Cannabis in 2009 and another 900 published in the first half of 2010 (according to a key word search on the search engine PubMed). **And what have we learned from these 20,000+ studies?**

• Cannabis and its active constituents are uniquely safe and effective as therapeutic compounds (unlike many over the counter meds).

• **Cannabinoids are virtually** non-toxic to healthy cells or organs**, and** incapable of causing the user to experience a fatal overdose **(like aspirin or opiates).**

• Cannabinoids do not depress the Central Nervous System. Therefore they possess a virtually unparalleled safety profile. Cannabis-based drugs were associated with virtually no serious adverse side effects in over 30 years of investigative use. (*CMAJ, 2008*)

Afraid of the High: *Science Daily (4/2009)*
U.S. and Brazilian scientists discovered:

> *the brain manufactures proteins that act like marijuana at specific receptors in the brain... discovery may lead to new marijuana-like drugs for managing pain, stimulating appetite, and preventing Marijuana abuse.*

BUT

> *Ideally, this development will lead to drugs that bind to and activate the THC receptor devoid of the side effects that limit the usefulness of Marijuana. Δ^9-Tetrahydrocannabinol (THC) exhibits anti-tumor effects on various cancer cell types, but its use in chemotherapy is limited by its psychotropic activity.*

(Lakshmi Devi, Mt. Sinai School of Medicine)

Afraid of The Paperwork:
Guzman cites a number of obstacles to human trials: including that cannabinoids are "still seen by many doctors and regulatory agencies as drugs of abuse," as well as **"lots of paperwork"** and a lack of commercial interest in natural compounds (can't be patented). "Cannabinoids have favorable drug-safety profiles. they do not produce generalized toxic effects of conventional chemotherapies. Cannabinoids are selective anti-tumor compounds, as they can kill tumor cells without affecting their non-transformed counterparts."

Why Not Combine Cannabinoids:
   (Like the real thing)
"Molecular Cancer Therapeutics:" Findings are the first evidence that combination cannabinoid therapy is more potent than ... just THC or other single cannabinoids "for glioblastoma and perhaps additional cancers:" "It is also possible that other constituents of Cannabis Sativa even those not structurally related to cannabinoids, such as **inert or inactive ingredients,** could improve the anti-tumor activity when combined." (McAllister)

Why Not Use The Whole Plant:
Smoked, vaporized, or an extract like Simpson's?

> *In regard to brain cancer, it is highly unlikely that effective concentrations of either Δ9-THC or CBD could be reached by smoking cannabis ...In regard to additional cancers, I feel defined formulations and dosing will be needed in order to effectively treat patients... team is moving toward clinical trials in both breast and brain cancer but it is a **slow process...** next step will be to try to replicate test-tube results in animals. No agency in the U.S. would allow me to move forward to clinical trials without some form of proof of concept data in a relevant preclinical in vivo model. (McAllister)*

It's Taking Sooo Long:
"Not only is there abundant evidence that cannabinoids kill cancer cells," (Armentano) "Investigators now even understand the mechanism of action; in other words, they know how and why cannabinoids kill cancerous cells and halt the spread of malignant tumors."

Redesigning the Cannabinoids:
Examining the effects of slight tweaks to the shape of a molecule is known as SAR for *Structure Activity Relationship*. While researchers at Organix did not comment on the recreational potential of their new chemicals, the SAR data shows that new drugs push the same pleasure buttons as THC and Anandamide.

Sitting on the Fence for Safety:
In *The Marijuana Cancer Cure Cult*, a liberal college professor who often advocates for Medical Marijuana, nevertheless echoes the nonsense that has held up relief for millions of patients and also encouraged the bias against the safety of the natural plant:

> *It's not as far-fetched as it sounds, but some enthusiasts* ***may be going too far!***
> (Mitch Earlywine, (Ph.D.)

He was referring to the largest and most respected study of its kind conducted by Kaiser Permanente in Oakland, California with 65,000 patients beginning in 1997 along with a **case-control study** (2006) in which patients with cancer were matched with patients without cancer (to compare risk factors) conducted through the UCLA Lab of Dr. Donald Tashkin, expert on pulmonary reactivity to drugs. He has been working with the government for years, attempting to validate deleterious effects of Marijuana on lung function and as a cause of cancer.

He failed every time to prove harmful effects of Marijuana with many studies over the years, but the conclusions of this last research was too stunning even for Tashkin. He has switched gears and become a guarded advocate of Marijuana as medicine. He has even made YouTube presentations to that effect.

Earleywine, usually considered an advocate for medical Marijuana, stresses that he is not dismissing the strong evidence that points to the possibility that some form of cannabis might be an effective cancer treatment: "*THC killing tumors is actually true*," **he says. "But we're not at human stage (of research)."** (NOT YET?) This was responded to by the famous Canadian who claims all sorts of cures with his oil from Marijuana flowers:

***Run From The Cure*:**
This is an amazing documentary of Canadian citizen Rick Simpson's experience with helping (curing) hundreds of Cancer victims with concentrated Marijuana flower oi. He is feared by the establishment and often referred to in derogatory terms and absolutely NOT taken seriously by the Medical Profession. He is painfully LOGICAL, outspoken and condescending to the medical critics who cite the lack of human studies that have been conducted with Cannabis.

"How are you going to do controlled studies when it is illegal in Canada to do so?" he said in an emailed response to questions. "As for possible risks (of his preparation which employs certain unhealthy solvents that are removed, of course, before any administration of his famous salve and which is displayed openly all over the internet, he argues, "*It is irresponsible to give people liver-toxic chemicals, chemotherapy and radiation, so if they (the doctors) are talking about irresponsible why not look at their own medical system?*

It is not irresponsible to save peoples lives (which Simpson is credited with having done by numbers of his patients themselves) *with a harmless natural, non-addictive medicine from nature. If you watch our documentary, you will see that I use a simple water purification process to get rid of solvent residue. I have been ingesting oil for over eight years and have supplied this oil to thousands of "cured people" for free.* http://topdocumentaryfilms.com/run-from-the-cure/

In an Interview with MND:
Al Byrne of *Patients Out of Time* said that the biological importance of Endo-cannabinoids in the human body are only now becoming known. For Byrne, new research is driving the bid to reschedule Marijuana: "There are more cannabinoid receptors in the brain and vital organs than any other receptor...The big discovery is that the human body is filled with cannabinoid receptors." **<www.medicalcannabis.com>**
.

Medical Conclusions: Data indicate that cannabidiol and possibly CANNABIS extracts enriched in natural cannabinoids are **promising non-psychoactive** anti-neoplastic strategies. In particular, for a highly malignant human breast carcinoma cell line, we have shown here that cannabidiol and a cannabidiol-rich extract counteract cell growth both in vivo and in vitro as well as tumor metastasis in vivo. Cannabidiol exerts its effects on these cells through a combination of mechanisms that include either direct or indirect activation of CB_2 and TRPV1 receptors and induction of oxidative stress, all contributing to induce apoptosis. BUT: **"Additional investigations are required!"** <http://www.medicalcannabis.com/Journal-2009/ama-and-medical-cannabis>

The News: The most recent cancer drug will cost about $100,000 per patient per year (2011), whereas: The cost of Marijuana for a cancer patient might cost close to $12,000 if purchased but probably would cost about $1000 if grown in the backyard. In addition, according to Guzman: *Cannabinoids have favorable drug-safety profiles and do not produce generalized toxic effects of conventional chemotherapies. (They) are selective anti-tumor compounds, as they can kill tumor cells without affecting non-transformed-counterparts.*

Humans are Marijuana Producers:

The War on Drugs has hit very close to home. Last year, scientists found that our skin makes its own Marijuana-like substance. Now, we see that our brain has been making proteins that act directly on the marijuana receptors in our head. The next step is for scientists to come up with new medicines that eliminates the nasty side of pot- a better joint, so to speak!

(Weissmann, M.D., The FASEB Journal)

Some Opinions and Facts:

*Since CBN and CBD don't have significant intrinsic activity on CB1 receptors ...do not produce psychotropic and **adverse side effects:*** (Felder, 1995)

Therefore: They are promising candidates as Anti-Inflammatory Therapeutics. (Showalter, 1996)

"modulation of the Endocannabinoid System will likely yield breakthroughs in the treatment of numerous, varied diseases and pathological conditions." From the *Journal of Pharmacological Reviews,* these conditions include:

> Mood and/or Anxiety Disorders; Movement Disorders, such as: Parkinson's and Huntington's Disease; Neuropathic Pain; Multiple Sclerosis; Spinal Cord Trauma / Injury; Cancer; Atherosclerosis; Myocardial Infarction; Stroke; Glaucoma; Obesity; Metabolic Syndrome, Hypertension and Osteoporosis.

Predictably, many patients who report experiencing therapeutic relief from Marijuana use it to treat symptoms or moderate progression of several of these same diseases. Cultural stereotypes and political biases against Cannabis and its active compounds should not impede the clinical investigation of Marijuana Therapy and its impact on this important biological system. Armentano:
<http://www.medicalcannabis.com/Journal-2009/ama-and-medical-cannabis>

Noteworthy:
~**Tylenol Pain Relief** comes from inhibition of FAAH which increases endogenous cannabinoids. Truth is that those who utilize Tylenol with all its dangerous side effects might much more safely employ Marijuana Therapy. Paracetamol or acetaminophen (in the U.S.) functions to inhibit FAAH. Subsequently, Anandamide levels in the body and brain are elevated. This action may be partially or fully responsible for the analgesic effects of acetaminophen ... cannabinoids, through an unknown mechanism and activates endogenous opioid pathways involving µ1 Opioid Receptor, precipitating dopamine release in the Nucleus Accumbens.

~ Cedaburg Hauser chemists have developed a process that **produces delta-9-tetrahydrocannabinol**, one of the most challenging members of the cannabinoid family...The process to produce multi-kilogram quantities of the key intermediate used in this process, which can be used to produce THC analogs as well, has been published by Cedarburg-Hauser scientists.

Pharmaceuticalizing Marijuana:
(Excerpt from Medican Interview)

GW is a Pharmaceutical Corporation that is developing a portfolio of *Cannabinoid Prescription Medicines* for a wide range of therapeutic conditions.

Med - Can one get High with Cannabis Medications?

GW - *By careful self-titration, most patients are able to separate the thresholds for symptom relief and intoxication, the 'therapeutic window', so enabling them to obtain symptom relief without experiencing a 'high'.*

Medcanaware - (Voice of Reason) "Patients' needs have been met for thousands of years by natural intact forms of marijuana ... range of conditions that natural Cannabis works for is far more than they are slowly starting to admit." Cannabis is the oldest medicine for true herbalists, who believe and apply only true herbs which are defined as "medicinal plants that are food first, then medicine, recreation and spiritual agents."

Med - Why Not just Let Patients Smoke Cannabis?

GW - In GW's opinion, SMOKING IS NOT acceptable delivery for a medicine.

Medcanaware Response - This may be true, although smoking herbs and other medicinal plant material have been applied as medicine for thousands of years. What about VAPORIZATION? (or) tea, yoghurt, cookies, cakes, salads, ice cream, you name it - it's a food first, then a medicine and recreant.

GW- We believe that patients wish to use a medicine that is legally prescribed, does not require smoking, is of guaranteed quality, has *been developed and approved by regulatory authorities for use in their specific medical condition and is dispensed by pharmacists under the supervision of their doctor.*

136

FYI - According to GW: In Canada, Sativex is marketed by Bayer Health Care. Once approved in the UK, Bayer will also market Sativex in that country. Upon approval in Europe (excluding the UK), Sativex will be marketed by Almirall. Upon approval in the United States, Sativex will be marketed by Otsuka.

Tragic Definition of Safe Medicine:
(According to Merck Institute, USA)
The main goals of drug development are effectiveness and safety. Because all drugs can harm as well as help, Ergo: Safety is Relative!!!! The difference between the usual effective dose and the dose that produces severe or life-threatening side effects is called the MARGIN OF SAFEY. The wider the margin of safety, the more useful is the drug.

BTW: Un-tampered with Cannabis (Herbal Marijuana which is not a drug) has a safety of **40,000 TO 1**, truly the most useful, safest herbal genus on earth.

Dr. Guy, U.K. - "Cannabis has the startlingly unusual property of being incredibly safe. The difference between a therapeutic dose and a deadly dose is 40,000. By comparison, the figure for aspirin is 25, while morphine is 50"

BUT WHEN IT COMES TO DRUGS - *Side effects are normal*, even if one of the side effects is death. *There is an 'acceptable' amount of deaths allowed in the Designer Death Drug Range.* (International Criteria of Harm and Safety), and *'acceptable' deaths can lead into the tens of thousands.*

End PART IV

Concluding Remarks (June 10, 2011)

The extent of the disservice that is being inflicted on the public by pharmaceuticalizing Marijuana cannot be overstated. Diminishing complex Cannabis molecules to one-directional synthetics indicates a deep ignorance of the Benefits of Marijuana. The living entity is an integrated holistic incorporation of constantly adjusting interconnections for maintaining balance. Intervention into such unimaginable energetic complexity with either an "upper" or "downer" is a foolhardy and arrogant oversimplification.

*The Marijuana Effect is classified as Neither Stimulant nor Depressant, but Both at the same time! which allows for an ever-adjusting equilibrium. The synergistic relationships of nearly 500 compounds that comprise the unique Marijuana plant cannot be replicated by science. Adding insult to injury: Not acknowledging the High of Marijuana that accompanies liberation in the breath/ freedom of the mind as the logical and proven **reliever of distress** makes poignantly clear that Drug Companies are at odds with the patient's well-being. That a flower can relieve the suffocation of years is too great a threat to be acknowledged by the profiteers. But it doesn't matter. With every formal study and through volumes of documented testimonials from around the world, it is undeniable: Marijuana Cures Cancer. The evidence cannot be hidden. It is out there in cyberspace for anyone who is interested. And more and more people are interested! Throughout this work, I have attempted to explain how the most basic effect of the magnificent Cannabis Sativa naturally dissolves the Cancer Biopathy through its unique compatibility with the human organism. Only a tiny sample of the volumes of specifics that support this fact have been offered, since again the precise information is written in cyber-space for anyone interested.*

Of course, there is additional evidence that I might have included to display even more intricate details of how Marijuana serves the body in its reversal of The Cancer Biopathy. Assuredly, over the course of future research, scientists will isolate yet more biological processes to determine exactly how the compounds of Cannabis Sativa interact with the human organism to facilitate health. For the purposes of this presentation, however, I think that the point has been made and the facts presented are sufficient. There should be no lingering doubt that Marijuana has an incredible synchronicity of action in the physical, psychological and spiritual dimensions of life. With wisdom, hopefully will come a modernized acknowledgement of natural and safe remedies unsullied by the profit motive. Perhaps this ancient plant which has travelled along the path of evolution with us and which has such a profound effect upon the consciousness of some receptive members of our race will contribute to a step up on the evolutionary ladder wherein there is realization that compassion and sharing are inherent to our actions rather than exploitation and self-concern.

The spiritual development that can be and very often is part and parcel of an ongoing association with Cannabis may help to raise the aspirations so that a new and higher plateau in personal understanding and motives may occur which is the only progression of any real significance. If the continuance of the human race is to have value from an esoteric point, only peace of mind and kindness of action will be deemed success.

The explanation of how Marijuana interfaces with the cells of the body to produce both physical and psychological benefits toward healing can be custom tailored to just about any chronic disease, with just the specifics being altered.

Also, many references concerning benefits that accrue from Marijuana are abbreviated since a fuller and integrated explanation is available in <u>The Benefits of Marijuana: Physical, Psychological and Spiritual</u>.

In referring to the spiritual aspect of a person, I realize that Science does not recognize such existence as necessary for the physical body, which is a direct, diametrically opposed viewpoint to the foundation of Holistic Health which accepts and reveres the reality that all manifestation is a reflection of the spiritual element whether we know it or not.

Questions from Readers:
I am happy to answer questions (without charge) about Marijuana for Cancer or any other health-related inquiries having to do with Marijuana.

In Friendship, Joan Bello
<http://www.benefitsofmarijuana.com/ask/ask-a-question/ >

There is no bibliography for this book. All studies cited are on the internet. The significance of the Pattern of the Breath for health and its integration with the workings of the body, mind and spirit is from my own personal knowledge/experience garnered from Yogic study.

Made in the USA
Charleston, SC
07 June 2014